Daktari Yohana

Daktari Yohana

An American Pediatrician in East Africa

John E. Hult MD

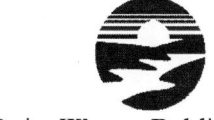

Quiet Waters Publications
Springfield, Missouri
1999

Copyright © 1998 by John E. Hult. All rights reserved. Printed in the United States of America. No part of this book may be used or reproduced in any manner whatsoever without written permission except in the case of brief quotations embodied in critical articles and reviews.

For information address Quiet Waters Publications, P.O. Box 4955, Springfield, MO 65808. E-mail: QWP@usa.net. For prices and order information visit:
http://ourworld.compuserve.com/homepages/QWP

Cover design by Myron Sahlberg.

ISBN 0-9663966-5-0

This book is dedicated to the memory of my parents,

Ralph and Gertrude Hult

whose love of, and respect for, the people of Africa
was constant and contagious,

and of our son,

Daniel Edwin Hult

whose vocabulary didn't include the word *stranger*,
and whose caring ways touched many lives,

and to

My medical co-workers

from Africa, Europe and America
with whom I was privileged to serve.

TANGANYIKA (in 1957)
Reference:
 Railroad ....
 Roads ____

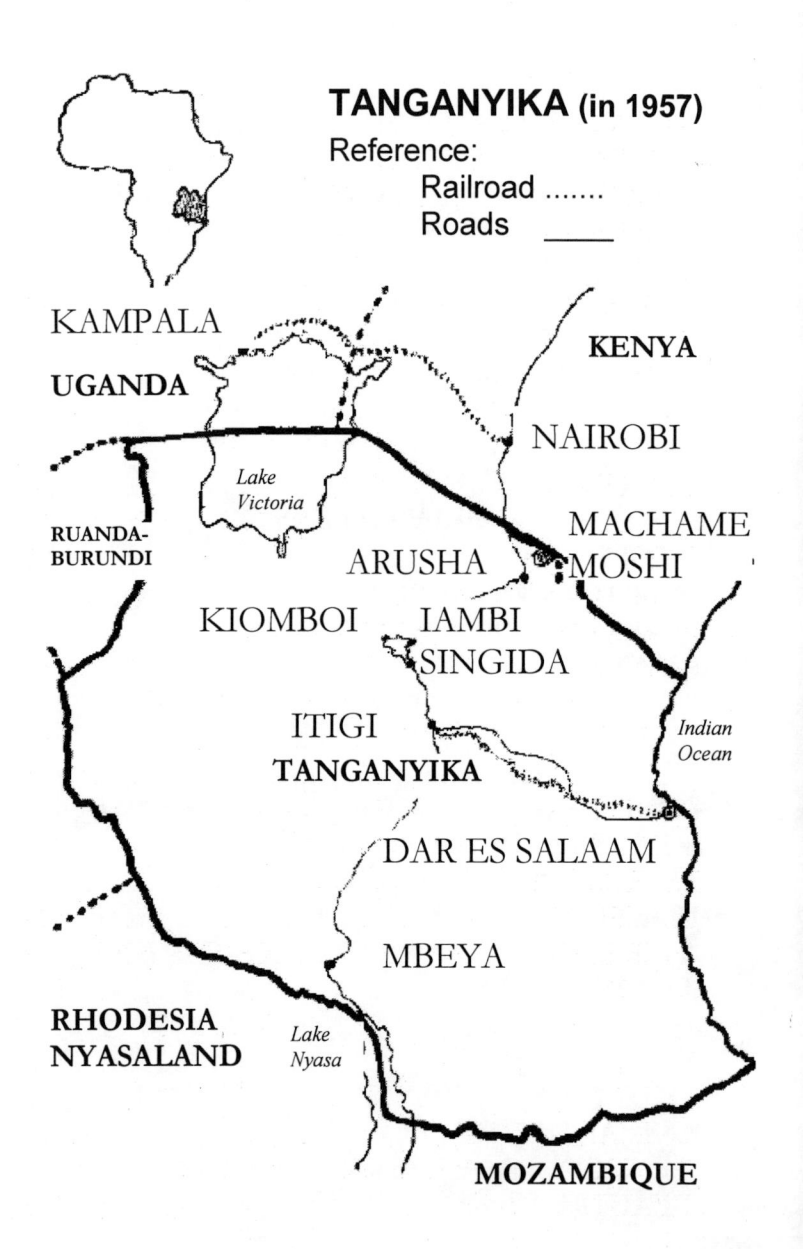

KAMPALA
UGANDA

KENYA

NAIROBI

Lake Victoria

RUANDA-BURUNDI

MACHAME
ARUSHA MOSHI

KIOMBOI   IAMBI
         SINGIDA

ITIGI
TANGANYIKA

Indian Ocean

DAR ES SALAAM

MBEYA

RHODESIA
NYASALAND

Lake Nyasa

MOZAMBIQUE

CONTENTS

1. FOREWORD 3
2. INTRODUCTION 5
3. "I CAN SEE! I CAN SEE!" 8
4. THE "MACHO" CLINIC 13
5. "HER HOUR IS AT HAND!" 18
6. "THERE ARE TWO POTATOES INSIDE YOU" . 25
7. "BUT THE BABIES WILL DIE IF THE MOTHER CAN'T NURSE THEM!" 30
8. "BUT EGGS ARE FOOD FOR OLD PEOPLE!" ... 36
9. AFRICAN MEDICAL COLLEAGUES 42
10. A DAY OF GREAT SORROW 51
11. "YOU TEACH ME YOUR MEDICINE AND I'LL TEACH YOU MINE!" 56
12. "AN EYE FOR AN EYE; AND A NOSE FOR A NOSE!" 61
13. POLIO COMES TO IAMBI 66
14. FEVER OF THE MOSQUITO 70
15. OUR YELLOW CHRISTMAS 75
16. "BUT DOCTOR! I NEED THE MEDICINE OF THE NEEDLE!" 79
17. "MY TOOTH HURTS!" 85
18. "WHEN ARE YOU GOING TO GIVE ME THE REAL TREATMENT?" 88
19. LEPROSY 93
20. UNWELCOME GUESTS 106
21. "HER BLOOD CELLS LOOK LIKE THE NEW MOON!" 113
22. MEDICAL EXAMINER FOR HER MAJESTY'S COURT 118
23. "THERE'S A LEOPARD IN MY HOUSE!" 123
24. ANIMAL DOCTOR 128
25. "HOW COULD YOU SHOOT THAT BEAUTIFUL CREATURE?" 133

26.	"SIAFU! SIAFU!"	139
27.	COBRAS, PUFF ADDERS, PYTHONS, AND MAMBAS	143
28.	AARDVARKS AND TERMITE TOWERS	148
29.	FEATHERED FRIENDS	154
30.	CAMPING WITH THE HIPPOS	159
31.	ADVENTURES IN THE SOUTHERN HIGHLANDS	164
32.	HAVEN OF PEACE	172
33.	LEARNING TIME IN KAMPALA	178
34.	ARUSHA, MOSHI, AND MACHAME	186
35.	SUNDAY MORNING MEMORIES	192
36.	EPILOGUE	197

1. FOREWORD

This book was written over several years through my participation in the creative writing class at the Chintimini Senior Center in Corvallis. My reference material has been personal journals, letters saved by our family, and medical records from our hospitals. These sources have jogged my memory to recall other experiences. Those of you who worked with me in Africa will undoubtedly remember some of them differently.

I have used place names as they were before 1961. For example, Tanganyika is now Tanzania. African personal names have sometimes been changed. We are now told that the correct spelling of Iramba is Ilyamba. The title of this volume DAKTARI YOHANA is the Swahili equivalent of "Doctor John."

Most of my medical activities involved the Iramba people but our mission also served the Turu tribe. For this reason I have sometimes used the term Iramba-Turuland when referring to our field of activity. We also cared for many people from the nomadic cattle-herding Barabaig tribe.

My stories focus largely on personal experiences. Little is said about the remarkable growth and vigor of the African church. We were inspired and enriched by our association with these vibrant first and second-generation Christians.

My special thanks are extended:

To Professor Simon Johnson and the members of our seniors' writing class who have endured all of these wild stories. They have constructively critiqued, encouraged and reacted. In every respect, they have been a wonderful support group.

To Roslyn Sadler and her late husband Dr. Wes, whose warm friendship and eloquent writings of their worldwide service have meant so much to Adeline and me.

To Dr. William Foege of Atlanta, Georgia, and Margaret Peterson RN, of Lindsborg, Kansas, who have reviewed my manuscript and made valuable suggestions.

To all of the members of our mission family who adopted us during our brief years in Tanganyika and continue to grow more like brothers and sisters to us as time goes by.

To many African friends who taught me more than I could possibly have taught them about faith, love, and healing.

To our five children for their special brand of love. All but Tim, who missed out on the African experience, have significant roles in several of these stories.

To my wife Adeline for her constant love and support. Without her patience, encouragement, constructive editing, and many hours at the computer, this volume would never have been completed.

John E. Hult MD
April 14, 1998

2. INTRODUCTION

The following stories have been written to record some of my experiences as a medical missionary in Tanganyika from 1957 to 1961. Most of these accounts grew out of medical adventures which were exciting and unique to a young pediatrician trained in the United States. Others relate to the fascination of living with my wife and children in a primitive land of awesome beauty and magnificent wildlife. I have focused largely on my own role in these events but much credit must be given to my coworkers from both Africa and America. I am deeply indebted to all the members of our mission family, most of whom have totally dedicated their lives in Christian service to Africa. Among them are some of my own personal heroines and heroes.

How did we get to Africa? For me it was actually a return trip. I was born in 1924 to missionary parents, Ralph and Gertrude Hult, in Old Moshi on the slopes of Mt. Kilimanjaro in Tanganyika. We had returned to America when I was two years old so I have no memories of that first African experience. I grew up hearing exciting stories about The Dark Continent with its fascinating people and their great needs. Initially, I wasn't driven by any great compulsion or calling to return to the land of my birth. I was strongly influenced by my father's return to Africa in 1942 and his death in Dar es Salaam less than a year later. I was deeply moved when my widowed mother volunteered for service as the matron of a mission orphanage in Bolivia in 1948. Additional inspiration came from my three sisters, Ingrid, Veda, and Eunice, who by 1953 were serving as missionaries in Cameroon, Tanganyika, and Pakistan.

My first wife Louise was a nurse. She and I seriously discussed working for our church in Africa at some time in the future. I was devastated by her untimely death in 1954. Our three children were only four years, two years, and seven months of age at the time. My dauntless fifty-five-year-old mother, home on furlough from Bolivia, came to the rescue. Her love, strong faith, and nurturing care enabled us to survive that crucial period. During the next few months, I became convinced that it was God's will for me to volunteer my services as a medical missionary to Tanganyika. The mission board accepted my application and agreed that Mother should go with me and the children if I wasn't remarried by the time I was ready to embark for Africa.

In order to be better prepared in adult medicine and surgery, I spent the next two years doing general practice with my uncle, Dr. Einar Norberg, in Cloquet, Minnesota. He had built Iambi Hospital to which I would be going and had worked there for fifteen years. He helped prepare me in many ways for the challenges I would face. I thoroughly enjoyed being a family doctor and had to exert a conscious effort not to put down permanent roots in this friendly community. Early in 1956 we moved to Minneapolis to make final preparations and to further my surgical training. To make ends meet financially, I was grateful for the opportunity to work part-time in the pediatric office of my good friend, Dr. Henry Staub.

Soon after this move I met a vivacious and attractive young lady named Adeline Lundquist. She was a missionary teacher home on furlough after serving four years in a Chinese Christian school in North Borneo. Our acquaintance blossomed into love. She already had her ticket to return to Borneo when she agreed to be my wife, the mother of my three children and to go with us to Africa. Our mission board executives agreed to this dramatic change of plans.

We were married on September 6th and honeymooned in New Orleans during the first trimester of my studies in tropical medicine at Tulane University. The urgent needs in Tanganyika prompted the mission board to request that we proceed to Africa after the second trimester. I could finish the nine-month course leading to a Masters Degree in Public Health and Tropical Medicine when we returned on furlough in four years. Accordingly, we made all of the necessary preparations, said our farewells to family and friends, and flew off to Tanganyika in April of 1957. Landing at the Nairobi Airport thirty-one years after our family's departure from Africa and being met by my sister Veda was an emotional experience, a symbolic spiritual homecoming.

My studies in tropical medicine were helpful, but it was impossible in a few months to absorb all the material and gain the skills to deal with the complex health problems of the tropics. I regretted my limited training and experience in surgery and obstetrics, knowing that I would often be confronted with overwhelming situations when working alone in Africa.

Four years is far too short a time to become familiar with the complexities of a culture totally different from ours. Our veteran missionaries told us that even after twenty or thirty years they were just beginning to be sensitive to subtle cultural differences. I was able to speak some Swahili, but not the various tribal languages. Having to work through interpreters, made it more difficult to function as a healer. For these reasons, many of the things I write in my accounts are subject to cross-cultural misinterpretations

In working with people on the other side of the globe, I was more impressed with how much we have in common than how much we differ. I grew to love and respect my African patients and fine dedicated medical coworkers. They helped to make those four years a special and cherished segment of my life.

3. "I CAN SEE! I CAN SEE!"

In May 1958 the monsoon rains had generously renewed the parched earth with life-giving moisture. The countryside around Kiomboi Hospital had been transformed from desert brown to a lush panorama of multiple shades of green. At the 5,000-foot altitude of the Iramba plateau, a gentle breeze moderated the 80 degree temperature to create a perfect sunny day.

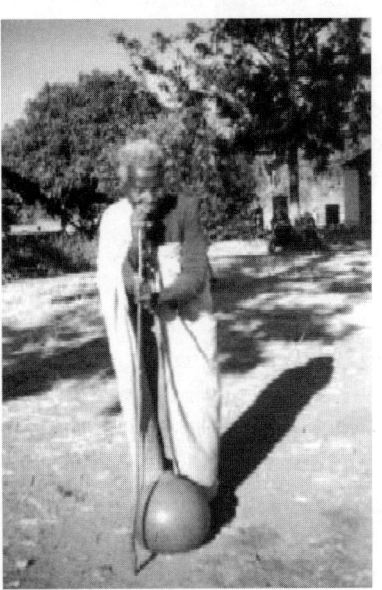

Blind Iramba widow

Late in the afternoon a small pedestrian caravan approached on the narrow sandy road. The column was led by several adults of varying ages. With fluid grace the women moved briskly along, balancing a variety of loads on their heads.

Perched delicately on the head of one young woman was a teakettle, a store-bought status symbol in this society.

Bringing up the rear was a small boy about six years old firmly holding the front end of a five-foot walking stick. Directly behind him, holding the other end of the staff, walked a spry little woman with snow-white hair. Barefoot and wearing only a loin cloth, the child was leading his blind grandmother in the traditional Iramba manner. (White canes aren't of much use in the African bush.) Welu and her family had arrived seeking help for her blindness. For nearly thirty years Kiomboi Hospital had been known as a place where eyesight could be restored.

The little group had walked for three days from their remote village over fifty miles away. No other transportation was available to them. Even if they had had a vehicle, the roads to their village were made impassable by the heavy rainfall on the sticky gumbo soil. This gummy, swampy terrain, known as mbuga, was almost impossible to traverse even with a 4-wheel-drive vehicle.

With one of our African nurses acting as interpreter, I interviewed and examined Welu. She was extremely alert and answered questions promptly and decisively. She spoke only Iramba, a melodious but very difficult tonal language. Welu understood virtually no Swahili, the lingua franca of Tanganyika, which was the only African language with which I had any familiarity.

Predictably, she was illiterate. There had been no schools nor any written words in the Iramba tongue when she was a child. Likewise, there were no calendars, so she knew neither the year nor the date of her birth. We were able to determine that she was at least seventy because she was already married and had given birth to two children by 1917 when the Wadachi (the German colonists) left. The year 1919 became the historic milestone during which German East Africa became the Protectorate of Tanganyika administered by Great Britain under the League of Nations. Even in remote areas, this event was well remembered by the Africans, including Welu.

She had given birth to nine children, five of whom had died in infancy or early childhood. She was now the matriarch of her clan, highly venerated and respected. Except for her close-cropped white hair and blindness, she appeared surprisingly youthful. Only a few wrinkles lined her ebony-hued skin. Her only garment was a black cotton sarong. Tribal markings tattooed her forehead and cheeks. She wore several strings of colorful beads around her neck. The soles of her bare feet were well protected by unbelievably thick calluses.

About twenty years earlier she had noticed difficulty in seeing the fine stems of grass with which she wove beautiful baskets. Since this was one of her special skills, losing this creative outlet was especially frustrating. Gradually she lost more vision. For ten years she had been so blind that she could only distinguish light and dark.

Using my ophthalmoscope, I determined that she had advanced cataracts with complete opacity of the lenses. Since this was a matter of great moment to all, we had a conference with all the members of her clan who had accompanied her. I indicated that we could almost certainly improve her vision with an operation. Both she and her family agreed that we should go ahead so we scheduled surgery for the following morning.

How does an American pediatrician acquire a skill as demanding and technical as cataract surgery? Before going to Africa I knew that this would be one of my responsibilities. There were no ophthalmologists in Tanganyika with its population of nine million. In apprehensive anticipation I had taken some training from a Minnesota ophthalmologist. In Africa I was fortunate to have the supervision of a doctor who had done extensive eye surgery in both China and Tanganyika. During my four-year term, I removed cataracts from over one hundred patients. In all but one of them, we saw significant improvement. That person had retinal disease concealed by the cataract.

In an ideal situation, we would do one eye and then wait until it healed to do the other. In Welu's case, we agreed to operate on both eyes on the same day because it was urgent that the family return home to plant their crops. If they waited much longer, there might not be sufficient food that year.

A smiling student nurse, attractively attired in a pin-striped green uniform, guided our patient into the women's ward and settled her into bed. Counter-pointing Welu's dark skin, the white hospital gown altered her appearance dramatically. She projected an almost regal aura as her family stood around her bed attending to her various needs.

Supper-time arrived. Actually, it was the only meal of the day for this Iramba family. Customarily at noon they drank a portion of magai, a slightly fermented non-intoxicating mixture of water and ground millet. We did not prepare meals for our hospital patients since most preferred to eat food cooked by their own families. Welu's daughter cooked a large bowl of ugali on an open fire in the lean-to kitchen behind the hospital. (Ugali is prepared by cooking cornmeal in water to a dough-like consistency.) Welu and her family gathered in a circle around the bowl. Very skillfully, each took a small portion, rolled it into a ball, and popped it delicately into the mouth. At home they would have had a side dish of meat and vegetables called mboga. This was eaten by making a hole in the ball of ugali with the thumb and scooping up some of the side dish. The Africans thought that our method of eating with knives, forks, and spoons was messy. Their mode certainly made dish-washing less complicated.

Soon after sunset Welu settled down for the night. Her daughter and grandson reclined on a grass mat under the bed. Unlike some families, they did not usurp the patient's bed. (On several occasions, while making night rounds, we would find our patient sleeping on the floor and a more privileged member of the family occupying the bed itself.) In spite of the eerie calls of prowling hyenas and night birds, everybody was soon fast asleep.

Early next morning Welu was given a mild sedative and taken to the operating room. Before surgery one of our nurses prayed aloud in Iramba that all would go well. As a recent Christian convert, Welu was visibly moved and responded with a very audible, "Amen!" I made the appropriate incisions under local anesthesia and removed cataracts from both eyes. During the surgery, she neither moved a muscle nor uttered a word of complaint. Both eyes were covered with protective dressings, sandbags were placed on both sides of her head, and the patient was returned to the ward.

Two days after surgery, with several of our staff in attendance, I removed Welu's bandages. Unaccustomed to the bright light, she blinked and tried to focus. One of the nurses, who had determined that Welu had never been near a white person, asked her; "What color skin does Daktari have?" Welu gently touched the skin of my forearm. Her eyes widened. "And what color is his hair?" the nurse continued. Welu hesitantly reached up to feel my mop of straight, bright red hair. After a brief pause and a look of astonishment, she exploded in a paroxysm of simultaneous laughter and flowing tears. We all laughed and wept with her.

She could see! She could see! With a little help from a pair of glasses, she could weave her colorful baskets again. With her walking stick, she could chase away hyenas who furtively attack blind elderly people. Maybe she would go to the new adult literacy classes and learn to read. Once again she could exult in the magnificent sunsets over the Rift Valley escarpment to the west of her home. For the first time she would be able to thrill to the bright smiles of her young grandchildren!!

4. THE "MACHO" CLINIC

A high percentage of people of all ages in the Third World suffer from disorders affecting their eyesight, most of which are preventable. It was particularly heart-rending to see children with impaired vision, and in pain, who could have been spared by simple measures. The Swahili word for eye is jicho which in the plural becomes macho. In our "Macho Clinic" at Kiomboi and Iambi Hospitals, we saw many patients with significant eye problems.

One day an anxious Iramba mother entered my office carrying her two-year-old son on her back. When she removed him from her kitamba (carrying cloth), I was horrified! His left eyeball was intensely inflamed and swollen, protruding an inch farther forward than the right. He was unable to close his eyelids, and his moaning cry indicated continuous pain. The normally transparent cornea was completely disintegrated. The lining of the eye became reddened a month earlier, with a slight discharge of pus. Each day there was more inflammation, swelling, and pain, but the family lived a two-days walk from the hospital and had no other access to medical care.

There was no hope of restoring function in the left eye. The right eye was becoming affected by a painful condition called sympathetic ophthalmia which would soon destroy its function if the damaged eye was not removed. I anesthetized him and carefully removed the eye, trying to preserve the muscles which move the eyeball so that an artificial eye might later be put in place. I tried unsuccessfully to use one of Dan's marbles to make space for a prosthesis. When our little patient awoke from anesthesia, the intense pain was almost completely relieved. We fitted him with an eye patch which made him look like an impish little pirate. How much better it would have been if we had seen him earlier and probably prevented the loss of his eye.

A few days later a young man came into the hospital with his left eye covered. He was in great pain. While out herding cattle, he had chased a calf out of the thick thorn brush into which it had wandered. A branch recoiled, impaling his eye with a two inch thorn. When I examined him, much of the fluid had been lost. All we could do was keep him quiet and protect him from infection. Fortunately, he did regain partial use of the eye. Time and time again, we saw people who had lost vision in one eye in the same way.

Albinos were another group of people who had serious visual problems. Several of them resided in our district. They suffered terribly in the bright sunlight, both from burned skin and painful eyes. With the absence of retinal pigment, they were often nearly blind. Sunglasses made them more comfortable but dimmed their vision even further.

One day when Martha was eighteen months old, we attended the African wedding of Wampumbula, a lovely young woman who had worked for us. Over one hundred people attended the feast after the ceremony. Among them was a little albino girl about ten years old, named Grace. She wore a black cotton sarong and covered her head and shoulders with a second dark cloth. When she spotted our little blondy, she was enthralled. Here was a child with the same pigmentation as hers! Grace wanted to touch and hold her, but Martha was terrified. She loved the dark-skinned friendly Africans and would have gone to any of them who reached out arms to pick her up. To her, the little black-shrouded albino appeared as a dreadful apparition. When Grace finally realized that Martha was afraid of her she was just crushed and nearly burst into tears. We tried to show our daughter what a neat little person was trying to befriend her, but she couldn't overcome her fear.

Every day we saw patients of all ages with trachoma, the leading infectious cause of blindness in the world. This insidious disease is caused by Chlamydia trachomitis, a bacteria previously thought to be a virus because it was so difficult to grow in the laboratory. When I hear the word trachoma, my memory screen flashes an image of an African toddler with a grimy face brushing pesky flies away from his (or her) runny eyes. That's when it all starts. No child escapes exposure to the infection, but those who have had the least contact with soap and water develop the worst disease. They keep re-inoculating themselves with obvious help from the swarms of flies. Studies show that thoroughly washing the face once a day significantly reduces the severity of trachoma. That is not easily accomplished when the mother has to walk miles to carry home the family water supply in a gourd on her head.

At first there is only slight inflammation of the lining of the eyes. Gradually this progresses to a thickened cobblestone appearance and an overgrowth of blood vessels onto the normally clear cornea. Even at this stage, treatment with antibiotic ointment cures the infection. Unfortunately, most of our population didn't have this option. As months and years go by, there is scarring and tightening of the tissues of the upper eyelids. This causes the coarse eyelashes to turn inward and scratch the cornea each time the eye blinks. Not only is this very painful, but within a few months the cornea becomes scarred and opaque with resulting blindness.

I'll never forget the first patient I saw with this devastating complication. She was an attractive middle-aged woman in obvious discomfort, squinting to protect her eyes from the light. Her upper lids were badly inverted and the eyelashes scraping the corneas. Whitish scars were forming where the coarse hairs abraded the surface so she was gradually losing her vision. My colleague, Dr. Viola Fisher, veteran of thirty years of medical work in China and Africa, had a solution. Under local anesthesia, she performed a simple operation removing a small wedge of tissue from the upper lid and sewing it back so the eyelashes were in a normal position. The patient was also treated with antibiotic ointment. She was delighted with the complete relief of her symptoms, returning in two months with normal vision. Later I did the same operation many times with similar gratifying results

At another hospital in Tanganyika, an unlicensed African medical worker had assisted doctors with this operation many times. He decided that he would do a little moonlighting, stole a set of instruments, went off into the bush, and set up his own little eye clinic. After he had done the operation on about fifty people, the medical authorities caught up with him. After checking his patients, they had to admit that his surgical technique was good. We didn't hear how he was disciplined, but his clientele considered him a true miracle worker.

Another significant eye problem resulted from Vitamin A deficiency. At the end of our seven-month dry season all green vegetation disappeared. The cattle foraged on brown dry grass and the chickens, likewise, had nothing green to eat. Adeline bought milk from our African neighbors, separated the cream, and churned butter. As the vegetation became completely dry, we were astounded to notice that the normal yellow color almost completely disappeared. It looked more like lard than butter. The yolks of the eggs also became almost white. When the rains came and green vegetation reappeared, the color returned to our butter and egg yolks.

In the late dry season, the human diet at Kiomboi was often deficient in Vitamin A. We saw babies and small children with dryness and thickening of the lining of the eyes. The more severe cases had softening and ulcers of the cornea. Without treatment this could rapidly proceed to permanent damage and loss of vision. A large injection of Vitamin A with adequate amounts to be given by mouth brought rapid healing unless the damage was already too extensive.

We tried to encourage people to provide for the dry season by having hand-watered gardens with green vegetables, yellow squash, pumpkins, and other Vitamin A producing foods. After we left Africa, I was pleased to hear that carrots, which grow well during the rainy season, have become popular in central Tanzania. Either fresh or dried, they provide an excellent source of Vitamin A in the diet. Improvements in nutrition and personal hygiene are still the most important steps in reducing the incidence of blindness in Africa.

My limited experiences as a macho doctor were gratifying, but I was terribly frustrated to see so much preventable blindness. Today, with limited resources, Tanzania is making significant progress in the prevention and treatment of eye disease. Much help comes from doctors and foundations in Europe and America in preventing and correcting visual disorders. The use of the airplane has enabled a handful of ophthalmologists with well-trained nurses and technicians to cover much of the country effectively. They have found that the most efficient use of funds involves teaching local medical workers and teachers simple measures to preserve visual health.

5. "HER HOUR IS AT HAND!"

The British Colonial Health Services issued a mandate in 1958 that we keep our medical records in English. Up to that time they had been recorded in Swahili, a language with which our African staff was much more familiar. The switch resulted in some interesting and sometimes amusing entries in the hospital charts. The medical assistants and nurses had studied English in school for a minimum of five years, but much of their English had been learned by reading the King James translation of the Bible.

One of our male nursing students was particularly imaginative in his use of English. In addition to his familiarity with the Bible, he eagerly latched onto American idioms, using them often. After his first day on duty in the obstetrical unit, we found the following entry in a patient's hospital chart:

"Her hour is at hand! Young maiden, great with child, admitted to the delivery room in deep travail, with much weeping and gnashing of teeth." After the patient delivered a healthy baby he wrote in the record: "Patient brought forth a son! Condition changed vice versa!" How could you say it any better?

To me, witnessing and participating in the miracle of birth has been one of the most exciting, gratifying, and renewing aspects of my professional life. Sharing the joy of a new mother holding her healthy baby in her arms for the first time is the stuff of which my most treasured moments have occurred. The Iramba patients loved their children dearly. Perhaps they cherished them in a way we don't fully appreciate because they were so vulnerable. At that time, the African mother knew that there was a fifty percent likelihood that her child would not survive to adult life. The rigors of tropical disease, malnutrition, and other forces beyond their control were devastating. We were there to teach that most of these threatening forces could be prevented or better controlled.

In the fifties, most Iramba mothers delivered at home. Unsanitary conditions and a lack of provision for complications led to a high maternal and newborn death rate. When she went into labor, a woman was usually attended by her mother, another close relative, or a village midwife. She was isolated in a separate room or hut. The presence of men was taboo. However, in extreme circumstances the medicine man might be called upon to divine which evil spirit was causing the problem. Delivery was accomplished from a squatting position on a dirt floor. Usually all went well, but if labor was prolonged or otherwise complicated, serious problems arose.

Difficult deliveries were not attributed to physical problems. They were considered to be the result of bewitchment or the intervention of ancestral spirits. The Mganga (medicine man) sometimes determined that the husband's seed was bad. One method of dealing with this problem was having the woman in labor drink a small amount of her husband's urine from a cow's horn poked through the wall of the hut in which she was in labor.

Forcefully binding the abdomen or pushing on the uterus was often tried late in labor. This definitely caused an increased incidence of uterine rupture. I heard a British government doctor lecture on a series of over one hundred women admitted with ruptured uteri to his hospital. He felt that pressure on the abdomen was a major cause of this complication. He even described one woman with a ruptured uterus who performed a Caesarean section on herself. In desperation, after many hours of labor, she opened her own abdomen with a knife. Since the baby, already dead, was free in her abdomen, she was able to remove it. Her family carried her to the hospital where the surgeon was able to repair her uterus. She survived and later had another baby in the hospital by Caesarean section.

Gradually the Iramba women learned that better solutions to difficult labor was provided in our hospital. Initially, only those with problems came, often too late. Soon after Kiomboi Hospital was built in the 1930s, several of the traditional midwives became convinced that the hospital was the best place to have babies. They persuaded the women of their villages to come, especially if they had had previous difficulties. One of these, Mama Salome, had joined the hospital staff over thirty years before my arrival. Two others joined her later.

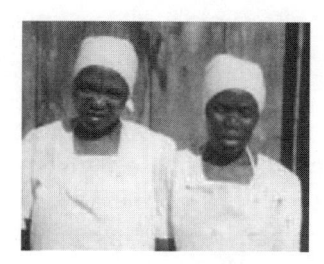

Iramba midwives

The midwives functioned primarily as interpreters, childbirth coaches, and surrogate mothers. The young Iramba women felt much more comfortable when the tribal midwives were present in the delivery room. They were able to calm those in distress and explain each aspect of the radically different environment. On one occasion, I heard Mama Salome tell an agitated young mother-to-be, "Now settle down! You're carrying on like an Mzungu!" (European woman). She had participated in the birth of three generations of babies and was one of our most respected and appreciated colleagues.

Our obstetric service was upgraded in 1958 when we replaced the small ward with a thirty-bed women's building.

Our well-trained American nurse-midwife, Greta Engberg, was joined by Christolumba, a lovely young Iramba woman who had graduated from our training school. Christolumba had then taken a year of midwifery training at a large obstetric service in Central Tanganyika. This capable team of midwives delivered most of the babies at Kiomboi. The doctors were called only when complications arose.

One of my most memorable obstetric experiences occurred at our fifty-bed hospital at Iambi. A young husband and members of his clan carried in his pregnant wife from a village several miles distant. She arrived on her wooden bed borne on the shoulders of four men of the family. She had been well until the day before when she suddenly collapsed while cooking supper. She complained of a severe headache and rapidly lapsed into unconsciousness.

When I examined this woman, about eight months pregnant, she was deeply comatose, barely breathing and totally unresponsive to any stimuli. It was obvious that she was dying. The most likely diagnosis was massive cerebral hemorrhage. With a stethoscope, I could hear two fetal heartbeats indicating that she was bearing twins.

We were totally unequipped for neurosurgery which probably wouldn't have saved her anyway. But we might be able to save her babies. When I presented this option to the father, his response was; "What's the use of saving the babies? They will die if their mother isn't there to nurse them." He had never known of a small baby who had survived its mother's death. Attempts to feed cow's milk had almost always ended in infant death. There was no woman in this clan who could wet nurse the babies.

After a lengthy conference, he was persuaded that we should try to save the twins. We volunteered to keep the babies in the hospital and feed them until they were at least six months old. We prepared the dying mother for surgery. Anesthesia was unnecessary. I performed a Caesarean section and delivered twin boys weighing four and a half and five pounds. The mother died several hours after surgery.

The twins were in poor condition. Our two American nurses took them home for the first few days and cared for them day and night. They fit snugly into a dresser drawer. When stronger and gaining weight, they were moved to the hospital. One of them subsequently died but the other went back to his family at six months.

Many other eventful obstetric experiences occurred. One dark night we were awakened by a commotion outside our bedroom window. A woman was obviously in distress. I hurriedly dressed, grabbed a flashlight and stepped outside. Two women were hovering over a third who was lying by the footpath to the hospital. Just as I arrived, I heard the lusty cry of a newborn baby. The young mother had started to the hospital just a little too late. We carried the patient with her healthy son on a stretcher to the obstetric ward. There were no complications. We were intrigued by the name which the family gave this little boy. Since he was born on the side of the path, they named him Njiani, which in Swahili literally means Along-the-trail.

Strong cultural beliefs were associated with the placenta in the old Bantu culture. The method of cutting the umbilical cord was considered important. One Ugandan tribe used a bamboo knife to sever a baby girl's cord and a sharp metal knife for that of a boy.

The Iramba tribal tradition prescribed that the placenta be buried, preferably on a river bank. A hole was dug the length of an arm and the cord suspended vertically so the end was near the surface when covered, supposedly to give the spirit an easier exit.

The placenta from twin births was often dried over a fire and placed in a gourd before burial. Parts of it were sometimes placed with grain seeds to insure a better harvest or given to goats to promote fertility.

When the dried cord came off the baby's navel it was tied to a string around the neck. We saw children as old as five years still wearing their mummified cords.

The occurrence of multiple births held a special spiritual significance in African culture. Many tribes feared that ancestral spirits were sending frightening messages through the birth of twins. In ancient times one or both babies were actually killed. One tribe in Northern Tanganyika was said to put twins outside, exposing them to wild animals at night. If the babies survived, they were considered special and nurtured carefully.

One young woman from a nomadic tribe delivered male twins at Kiomboi hospital. We soon noticed that the mother was only nursing the firstborn. Our nurses spent much time and effort in persuading her to feed the other one. By the time of discharge she seemed to have bonded with both twins. The second-born was nursing hungrily and gaining weight, but we still had grave concerns about his future.

Mama Salome informed us that the birth of twins had usually been a good omen in the Iramba tribe. We witnessed happiness about multiple births among both Christian and non-Christian parents. I was introduced to a young mother at the Wembere dispensary with beautiful happy six-month-old twin girls. Interestingly they were named "Bibi Veda" and "Mama Maria" after my sister Veda and the Iramba midwife who had delivered them. All signs indicated that they were cherished and loved by their families.

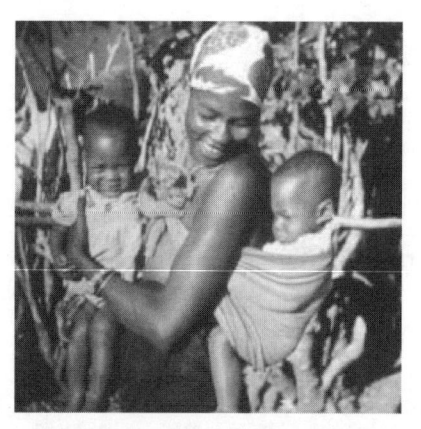

Twins Bibi Veda and Mama Maria

We mission doctors considered delivery of the babies of our American co-workers to be a special privilege. Each arrival was greeted with joy and excitement by the entire mission family. Dr. Viola Fisher delivered most of the little ones on our Iramba-Turu area until her retirement. In one year she ushered six new "nieces and nephews" into the world, including our daughter Martha.

Dr. Joe Norquist delivered the premature daughter of Shirley and Doug Augustine. Cindy required special attention. Her inventive father constructed a marvelous little incubator from some of his photo-developing equipment. She thrived! A week later, I delivered another preemie, Joyce, to Bev and Dave Henry. Anxious moments followed as Bev hemorrhaged after the delivery. She needed a transfusion but no one with compatible blood was available. Just at that moment Doug Augustine drove in from Kinampanda, twenty miles away, to visit his wife and daughter. He was the only one we knew with Type O-Rh negative blood. The cross-match with Bev's was perfect and he was quickly pressed into service for a transfusion. After a few scary moments, Bev went on to a happy recovery. Joyce also grew and flourished after early feeding problems.

Why had Doug come along at just the right time with his special life-sustaining gift? Miracles still happen and our prayers are answered.

6. "THERE ARE TWO POTATOES INSIDE YOU"

The birth of a healthy baby brought great happiness and fulfillment to an Iramba woman, her family and her clan. Not being able to have children was a tragedy. Having many babies compensated for the high childhood mortality. Only five of every ten babies born in our area could be expected to reach adult life. In the old tribal culture, barrenness was a legitimate reason for divorce. The health and strength of the tribe depended upon the fertility of the women. The possibility of male sterility was not often considered even though it was responsible for half of the childless marriages.

At Kiomboi Hospital we conducted a weekly women's clinic. At each session we examined up to one hundred women. Most were concerned about fertility, although none would initially verbalize that reason for their presence. Their first words were almost always, "Kiuno kinauma." (My lower back hurts.) We therefore called this weekly session our KK clinic. No doubt low back pain often occurred, but it wasn't the primary reason for the visit. It seemed to be the socially acceptable way to approach the doctor.

We discovered that the main concern was inability to conceive or to carry a pregnancy to term. Many had abnormalities which we were unable to correct. Pelvic inflammation was common with tubal blockage often caused by venereal disease or sometimes by genital tuberculosis. A small percentage of our patients were found to have ovarian cysts and other masses which we could surgically remove.

When we did surgery, the family members were always anxious to see what we had taken out. On one occasion I excised a softball-sized dermoid cyst from a woman's ovary. This particular tumor originates when an immature egg cell multiplies in an uncontrolled reproductive surge. This usually benign growth is made up of hair, teeth, and other skin related tissue. When I showed this grotesque mass of kinky hair and well-formed human teeth to the family, they were initially speechless but then greatly relieved that it was no longer inside her. No doubt they speculated about what kind of a mysterious and powerful spirit had invaded her. They did seem satisfied that our intervention had cured her, but I suspect that the medicine man was also consulted and that certain evil spirits were exorcised.

One day I checked a woman who had suffered five miscarriages, all at about five months. That was an unusual time for spontaneous loss of a pregnancy. When I examined her internally I was astonished to find a double uterus. I had never seen this abnormality except in textbook illustrations. In my excitement, I hastily tried to explain the situation to her. It so happens that the Swahili word for uterus is kizazi and for potato it is kiazi. This class of nouns is pluralized by substituting vi- for ki-. I had never used the plural for uterus before, so my Swahili sentence came out, "Una viazi viwili ndani!" (You have two potatoes in here.) The poor woman was horrified. The African nurse laughed heartily and corrected my mistake, "Una vizazi viwili ndani!" Apparently neither of her vizazi was developed enough to sustain a pregnancy for nine months. Unfortunately, there was nothing we could do to correct this major problem.

Another fairly common occurrence was tubal pregnancy, which often resulted from previous infection, scarring, and blockage of the tube from the ovary to the uterus. Afflicted women were brought in to the hospital after the growing embryo ruptured the tube, causing life-threatening internal bleeding. After missing at least one menstrual period, the patient would experience severe lower abdominal pain on the affected side, then gradually show symptoms of anemia and shock from internal bleeding. A tentative diagnosis was made by inserting a long needle through the vagina behind the uterus and finding dark blood in the abdominal cavity. In one sequence, while I was the only doctor at Kiomboi Hospital, I diagnosed and operated on three of these cases within a four-day period. In each, the tube was ruptured with embryos at the two-month stage outside the tube but within the abdominal cavity. After removal of the damaged tubes, all three of these patients recovered rapidly and completely.

Some exciting events occurred on the day of the third case in this series. The young woman was carried in by her family late in the afternoon with a typical history. My examination indicated bleeding into the abdomen, which made the diagnosis almost certain. She was not in shock so, while she was being prepared, I hurried home for a quick supper. Just as I arrived at our house, a jeep drove up and an elderly man stepped out. He introduced himself as Dr. Brown, a retired gynecologist from Texas. He was unofficially visiting mission hospitals all over Tanganyika. Adeline invited him in to have supper with us. While eating, I told him about our impending emergency surgery. Knowing that this was his specialty, I invited him to do the surgery with my assistance. First he asked, "What makes you so sure this is a tubal pregnancy?" When I reviewed our findings and told him that this was the third case in four days he was astounded. In the last ten years of his practice in Texas, he had operated on only one case. He insisted that I do the surgery and that he be the assistant. We finished our hasty meal and hurried to the hospital.

By then it was completely dark. Just as we reached the hospital, the medical assistant assigned to the surgical team came dashing up as fast as he could run. He was trembling, terrified, and almost incoherent. When he had partly regained his composure, he managed to explain his fright. Just as he had left his house not four hundred yards away from the hospital, he had heard a nearby hyena emit the unique and eerie call which was associated with death. In the folklore of the Iramba people it meant that somebody in the vicinity was soon going to die. We tried to reason with this bright educated young man, but he was still so shaken that it was obvious he would not be able to perform his duties. He seemed relieved when I excused him and sent him home, escorted by a nurse with a lantern. Dr. Brown shook his head in amazement.

By then all was in readiness for surgery. Using ether, our nurse anesthetist soon rendered the patient unconscious and I proceeded to open the abdomen. It was filled with dark blood. We found the right Fallopian tube ruptured with the well-formed embryo plainly visible. Just at that moment a hyena laughed noisily right outside the open operating room window. Dr. Brown jumped and blurted, "What was that?" What little we could see of his face blanched to the color of his white surgical cap and mask. We hastened to reassure him that it was just a hungry hyena investigating the smell of blood. As he recovered his composure, he chuckled nervously. Gradually his color returned. After we had finished surgery and saw that the patient was in good condition, he exclaimed, "Wait until my friends back in Texas hear about my evening at Kiomboi Hospital!! They won't believe it!!"

Our patient was unaffected by the evil spirit of the hyena. As I made rounds the following morning, she smiled and asked when she could return home.

One of our encounters in the KK Clinic had a happy ending. The Barabaig tribe, a nomadic cattle-herding people, occupied territory adjacent to Irambaland. A sub-chief brought in his tall and comely daughter who appeared to be in her early twenties. She wore a beautiful calfskin dress colorfully embroidered with fine beads. Her forearms and lower legs were heavily decorated with brass ringlets. She walked with a stately graceful gait. By any standard, she was a strikingly attractive young woman, but she appeared to be very depressed. The primary concern was that she had never had a menstrual period although she was at least five years past the age when this should have occurred. Until this biological landmark was reached, she was ineligible for marriage.

In my examination, I first noted that her lower abdomen was enlarged to about the size of a four-month pregnancy. Then I discovered that her vagina was covered by a thick tough hymeneal membrane. Clearly this was the cause of her problem; the swelling of her tummy was the result of trapped secretions from her uterus. I explained to her and her father that we could indeed help her with a simple operation. With their consent, I made an opening in the membrane under local anesthesia. At least a quart of liquid secretions drained out and the swelling of her lower abdomen disappeared. After a day in the hospital she was discharged with instructions to return in three months.

When that time had elapsed, she and her father reappeared, both smiling broadly. She had had two monthly periods and her father had contracted a marriage with an eligible young man for an unspecified number of cattle. As her father related the details, she smiled coyly and hid her face in her hands.

7. "BUT THE BABIES WILL DIE IF THE MOTHER CAN'T NURSE THEM!"

Soon after beginning work in Tanganyika I came to the conclusion that breast feeding was almost as critical to our African babies' welfare after birth as the umbilical cord was before they came into the world. Over and over again we heard the stories of small babies perishing after the mother's death or serious illness. The young father I told about in an earlier chapter was reluctant to give his permission to try to save the twins when his wife was dying. Several times he repeated his argument, "But the babies will die if the mother can't nurse them!" The survival of a tiny baby whose mother had died was unbelievable. When he finally consented and we did manage to deliver his sons alive, he was delighted. The principal reason for these double tragedies with loss of both mother and baby arose from the near-total failure of artificial feeding.

If the mother or another woman in the family couldn't nurse a baby, efforts were made to feed the infant cow's or goat's milk. In most of Africa there is no refrigeration and no availability of bottles in which to prepare and store formula. At Iambi Hospital, I was horrified to witness a woman from a nomadic cattle-herding tribe, trying to 'bottle feed' her three-month-old nephew whose mother had just died. She poured sour milk from a gourd into the palm of her hand held next to the baby's mouth, trying to force the liquid in. As the little tyke struggled and spit it out, she held it up over his nose. He coughed and sputtered, probably drawing some into his lungs. Since he was very hungry, he eventually took several handfuls with a lot of choking and gagging. Many of the babies fed in this way no doubt died of aspiration pneumonia. I never saw such drastic force-feeding by our Iramba mothers, but most of those with whom we talked felt that practically all of the babies who couldn't be nursed by their mothers or a family member would die.

When a mother died in our hospital and there was no relative to breast-feed the baby, we kept the infant in a small separate ward for the first few months. We assigned African nurse's aides to care for such orphans day and night. At times we had as many as six of these infants in our care. Our missionary nurses supervised the preparation of formula and the total care of our charges. More often than not, they were the ones doing most of the night-time care and feeding. Our American nurses frequently took the tiny and sickly orphans into their own homes until they were stronger.

We dreaded sending these babies home after six months. By then we were quite attached to them. We knew that, even with loving families, their mortality rate would still be terribly high. They did not have the protection from breast milk antibodies nor the cleaner environment of the hospital.

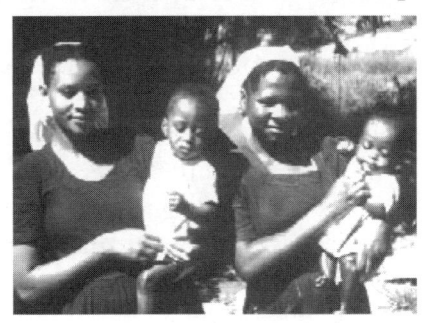

Orphans with nursing aides

In more urban areas the abandonment of breast feeding in favor of the bottle created another set of problems. In 1960 I attended a World Health Organization conference on tropical child health in the large city of Kampala, Uganda. As I was riding on a bus through dismal slums on the outskirts of the city, I saw a full-sized billboard portraying a radiantly healthy smiling African baby with a bottle. The huge caption proclaimed, "Strong As Iron!" This attractive display, which advertised one of the major cow's milk formulas, had a powerful appeal to the mothers who wanted only the best for their babies. My reaction was that these oversized public documents could lead inadvertently to the death of thousands of little ones.

The international authorities at the conference confirmed that impression. Dr. Hebe Welbourne's research in Kampala indicated that serious life-threatening diarrhea occurred four times more often in bottle-fed babies than those nursed by their mothers. The death rate from diarrhea was highest in the poorer sections of the city. Breast milk has been shown to promote the growth of friendly bacteria and to inhibit the growth of those causing infections. It contains one type of the mother's antibodies which transmit to the baby some of her own body's germ-fighting wisdom. Breast-fed babies also have a lower incidence of iron deficiency anemia. These are but a few of the factors which mandate breast feeding in an environment with so many obstacles to childhood survival.

In rural Irambaland we didn't have to worry about the encroachment of the almighty bottle. There really wasn't any viable alternative to breast-feeding. Most of the missionary wives nursed their babies, reinforcing the African mothers' awareness that this was the best way to feed a child.

After we left Africa, one of the Kiomboi missionary wives, Annette Stixrud, was nursing her son who was only a few months old. An African pastor's wife was so ill after a difficult delivery that she couldn't nurse her newborn. Her husband came to Annette assuming that she would have some formula bottles he could borrow to feed his baby girl. She said, "No, I don't have any bottles, but I can nurse her along with my son until your wife is stronger." For two weeks she nursed both babies day and night until the African mother was well enough to take over again. We have heard that this same little girl still keeps in touch with her American 'surrogate' mother and that she will soon graduate from the University in Dar es Salaam. Annette admits to being taken aback when the father introduced her as "my daughter's mother."

Sometimes breast-feeding wasn't easy. One day a young mother with a tiny baby boy came to my office. When she undid her sarong to show me her problem, I was shocked. A tropical ulcer had invaded and destroyed all the skin of her left breast except for a circle about an inch in diameter around the nipple. Tropical ulcers are caused by an infection which slowly eats away all layers of skin. Here was an angry open sore five inches in diameter. This courageous woman was, with much painful effort, still nursing her baby on this side. The right side alone didn't satisfy his lusty appetite.

I consulted with another mission doctor. His initial reaction was that a mastectomy with removal of the entire breast was the proper approach and would give her immediate relief. I argued that I would like to attempt a skin graft first. We had had good success in grafting tropical ulcers. Most of them had been on the lower legs, some as large as this one on the breast.

We admitted our patient to the hospital, cleaned up the ugly ulcer and treated her with large doses of penicillin. Then I carefully covered the entire ulcer with thin strips of skin taken from the inner thighs with a straight razor. (We didn't have a fancy machine to precisely prepare our skin grafts.) We gently bandaged her breast and told her that her hungry son would have to be satisfied with the right side for the time being. He wasn't happy about going on 'half-rations.'

Three weeks later I was pleased to find that all the grafts had grown in place so she was able to carefully start nursing again. After six weeks all was healed and no breakdown had occurred. The end result wasn't esthetically attractive but the breast was completely serviceable. She clearly indicated her gratitude and so did her young son. She even said that he liked the breast that we had fixed up better than the other.

On several occasions I witnessed grandmothers consoling unhappy babies by putting them to the breast. At first I thought that they did so purely for pacification. Most of the time that was true, but one day a pleasant woman with streaks of gray in her hair saw me watching her nursing a baby which I knew was her granddaughter. She smiled as she demonstrated to me that there was a small drop of milk coming from the nipple. She said, "Kidogo tu!" In Swahili that is to say, "Just a little bit." Many examples prove that a woman can put a baby to breast and initiate lactation if she has the will and the patience. Mama Salome told us that she had known several women who hadn't had babies for several years begin to produce milk again. She emphasized that they had to be patient and put the baby to breast frequently. They also tried to obtain a supply of special nuts which were thought to stimulate the flow of milk. The success of these heroic measures could be life-saving for a baby who couldn't be nursed by the mother.

One of the most significant benefits of breast-feeding in the Third World has been its effect of delaying the next pregnancy. As long as a mother is nursing several times daily there is a high level of the hormone prolactin which inhibits the release of egg cells from the ovary. It is not a sure-fire method of birth control but greatly reduces the percentage of women who conceive.

In many of the tribal cultures, sexual intercourse was taboo as long as the mother was breast feeding. With polygamy this was acceptable to the husbands but that changed with the widespread adoption of monogamy. The women of the three tribes among whom we worked all nursed their babies until they were from fifteen to eighteen months old. Our monogamous Christian mothers had abandoned the taboo on sexual intercourse while nursing, but still the pregnancies were spaced very close to two years apart. In urban areas, many monogamous women who had adopted bottle feeding began having babies every year.

I have many pleasant memories of African mothers nursing chubby healthy babies. One that particularly stands out is that of the blind mother who was brought to me by her husband in the hope that we would be able to fix her bad eyes. Robust twin boys, about five months old, were slung securely on her back in a brightly colored cloth. I seated her on a chair in my office and did a brief examination as her husband stood beside her. Both of her eyes were scarred and shriveled beyond any hope of repair. As I explained this to the young couple, sadness was reflected in their faces.

Then one of the twins cried and the other squirmed vigorously. With smooth practiced motions the mother released her carrying cloth and positioned her sons so that each was able to hungrily latch on to one of her breasts. Her husband gently placed his hand on her shoulder to help her assume a less awkward posture. The expression on her face became one of calm acceptance and she smiled briefly in my direction. One of the babies eyed me suspiciously but kept on sucking vigorously. His brother buried his face in his mother's breast and emitted a veritable symphony of contented gurgles and grunts. She may have been visually handicapped, but her sons eloquently informed us that she was still a terrific mother! Those little boys, and thousands of other bright healthy ones like them, convinced me that breast-feeding was the only way to go in Africa.

8. "BUT EGGS ARE FOOD FOR OLD PEOPLE!"

Every year millions of children around the world die from malnutrition. Almost daily we are confronted with television and newspaper images graphically depicting the horrors of childhood starvation. In Africa we lived in an area which received adequate rainfall and was not overpopulated. In the absence of war and famine we saw relatively few cases of malnutrition. When these did occur, the problems usually resulted from failure to use available foods because of misinformation and tribal taboos.

One morning at Iambi Hospital, I spotted a young Iramba mother seated in the waiting area of the clinic holding her two sons. One was a robust healthy two-month-old infant, vigorously nursing at her right breast. With her left arm she cradled 'big brother,' a two-year-old boy named Makala, who projected an image of abject misery as he whimpered weakly and irritably. His skin was much lighter than his brother's and his hair nearly blonde. I immediately recognized that here was an urgent situation. This was the first case of serious protein malnutrition, commonly known as kwashiorkor, which I had ever seen. The child was dangerously ill so we admitted him directly to the hospital.

The concerned young mother gave us the following story of Makala's life: He was her firstborn, starting out as a chubby dark-skinned baby who looked much like his new brother. There was plenty of milk in her breasts and Makala was blessed with a lusty appetite. By one year of age, he was a fat happy child who walked and was starting to talk, dance and sing. The mother became ill with malaria and gradually lost much of her milk supply. She nursed Makala less and less but continued until he was about eighteen months old, when she discovered that she was pregnant.

The mother abruptly weaned him and turned him over to her twelve-year-old sister who cared for him most of the time. This freed up the mother so she could more easily cultivate her garden, carry water from the river a mile away, cook for the family, and do the laundry. Makala liked his aunt but was quite unhappy that his mother had virtually abandoned him. He lost his appetite for the only foods provided him, bananas and a gruel made from ground corn. He was often sick with fever and diarrhea and began losing weight. Although the family had an available supply of milk, eggs, and peanuts he received none of these high-protein foods. When I asked the mother about eggs, she appeared surprised, and replied, "But eggs are food for old people!"

Since Makala was weaker, she felt that he should only have the light foods. For over six months he had existed on a diet which was terribly deficient in protein. Now that he was sick, the concerned mother devoted more time to him, but his condition deteriorated further when the new baby arrived. The family was shocked to see the color of his skin and hair fading until he was almost white. His personality transformed from that of a happy outgoing child into a cranky little old man. No longer did he walk or play or laugh. When he began to have difficulty breathing, he was brought to the hospital.

When I picked Makala up and put him on my lap to examine him, I was horrified. His feeble shrill cry reminded me of a tiny bird. He resented my intrusion, but his wasted muscles were too weak to push my hand away. The normal layers of baby fat had disappeared to be replaced by fluid under the skin, known medically as edema. My fingers with only slight pressure left deep imprints on his legs and arms, just as if I had squeezed a piece of modeling clay. His breathing was labored, and I could hear lung sounds suggestive of pneumonia. The abdomen was bloated. A blood test showed that he was anemic. The outer layer of skin on his thighs was peeling like paint off an ancient building. His skin was the color of old ivory and is hair quite blond.

Makala was able to take fluids by mouth so we began giving him a dilute skim-milk formula every three hours. His pneumonia was treated with antibiotics and liberal doses of vitamins. He took his feedings poorly, but at the end of the first twenty-four hours the intake was adequate. He seemed slightly improved and we took him outside to take his picture. That night at ten o'clock rounds we found the mother and her two little boys sleeping quietly together in one hospital bed. About midnight the nurses were startled by screams coming from the children's ward. Makala was found dead in his mother's arms! I was called immediately and hurried to the hospital. Knowing that severe kwashiorkor has a terribly high mortality rate wasn't reassuring at all. I blamed myself for not being more alert to the seriousness of his condition, but there was little more that we could have done.

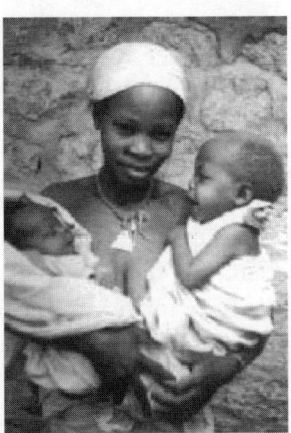

I saw a total of about twenty children with kwashiorkor. In spite of our efforts, three of them died soon after admission to the hospital. Most were between eighteen months and three years of age with histories very similar to that of little Makala. I can't remember a single case in which protein-rich foods weren't available in the home of the afflicted child. Certain high-protein foods, such as eggs, simply weren't being used because of cultural taboos.

One little girl two years of age fit the classical picture of the so-called sugar baby protein malnutrition. She had been given plenty of carbohydrates but virtually no protein for several months. She was quite chubby with fat little cheeks, but was irritable and lethargic. Her skin and hair had bleached dramatically. Her muscles were so weak that she couldn't stand alone. The family was excited and delighted to recognize her improvement after milk and ground peanuts were added to her diet.

The term kwashiorkor was introduced in 1935 by Dr. Cicely Williams, widely revered as "the mother of tropical pediatrics." She was working in the Gold Coast of Africa and heard the Accra people use kwashiorkor to describe a condition identical to that of Makala. The term literally means the disease a child gets when the next baby is born. It is not confined to Africa and is just one of the extreme variants of protein malnutrition. Those who recover usually have some degree of permanent brain damage.

Depigmentation of skin and hair is the most startling feature of kwashiorkor. Imagine how alarming it would be to witness your beautiful dark-skinned child's color fade away. If I had been an African parent, I would have been convinced that evil spirits were operating. The simple explanation is that the protein intake is so limited that there isn't enough of the one specific amino acid from which the dark pigment melanin is derived. You can't paint a house black without some black paint. Dark skin is vital in sunny climates as a protection from intense solar radiation, and to limit the production of too much Vitamin D. Conversely, light skin is advantageous in temperate cloudy climates to capture scarce ultraviolet rays to synthesize that same Vitamin D.

Kwashiorkor occurs throughout the world, especially in developing countries. In 1969 I saw more cases in three weeks in Honduras than I had observed in four years in Africa. Depigmented hair colors vary with different ethnic groups. Affected Asian children tend to have red hair instead of blond. In my tropical medicine class at Tulane University in 1956, I studied with five young doctors from Indonesia. They had flown directly from Djakarta to New Orleans so I was the first adult they had ever seen with red hair. They told me that they were at first alarmed, thinking that I must have a serious protein deficiency. The only human hair like mine which they had previously seen had been on children with kwashiorkor. I convinced them that I consumed adequate amounts of protein, but I still wasn't out of the woods. One of them laughingly told me that my hair color was also identical to that of the great ape known as the orangutan. The thought had crossed his mind that I might be closely related to that old man of the forest. It's not easy for us redheads to command respect!

My limited experiences in Tanganyika pale in comparison with the massive starvation occurring in the world today. Even here in America there are far too many children with dietary deficiencies of protein and other nutrients. Sadly these are often the result of carelessness, indifference, neglect and ignorance. If we could only invest a small fraction more of ourselves and our resources in the total welfare of children, the world would profit immensely.

One of the most encouraging advances in the battle against protein malnutrition has come in the field of plant genetics.

Nobel Prize Winner Norman Borlaug developed a species of maize (corn) which contains all of the essential amino acids. When introduced in Third World countries, whose staple diet is mostly corn, malnutrition is dramatically reduced.

Dr. Bill Foege, a world-renowned public health crusader, was one of the principal leaders in the conquest of smallpox. I have been in touch with him since 1963 when he was a public health officer in Denver and I was the pediatrician for his young son. He has reviewed my African stories and wrote on June 25, 1997:

"Your mention of Dr. Cicely Williams brought many memories. Years ago I had dinner with the head of state of Ghana, Jerry Rawlings, President Carter, and Nobel Prize winner Norman Borlaug. We were urging Rawlings to help introduce a new strain of maize that has all the essential amino acids. I mentioned that Cicely Williams had introduced the word 'kwashiorkor' to the world from Ghana and that it would be nice if the solution also came from Ghana in her lifetime.

"Rawlings asked me, 'Is she still alive?' I answered, 'Yes,' and he asked, 'How old is she?' I said she was ninety-five. He sat bolt upright and said, 'We don't have much time!' He asked Dr. Borlaug if he could have a plan by the next morning. By the time she died at age ninety-eight, we were producing the new corn and it was being sold as a weaning food. Borlaug and I returned last year to find that 40% of corn grown in Ghana is now of the Quality Protein variety. Malnutrition is declining but no one even notices."

9. AFRICAN MEDICAL COLLEAGUES

We American doctors and nurses realized that the most significant part of our medical program should be the motivation and training of indigenous health care providers whose work would continue after we returned home. I cherish the memories of personal and professional interaction with African dressers, nurses, midwives, and medical assistants. In many ways I gained and learned more from them than they did from me.

When our first medical missionaries came to Irambaland about 1930, only a handful of Africans could read and write and none was familiar with Western medicine. The doctors and nurses began by recruiting bright young men called dressers for on-the-job training in the clinics and hospitals. They were taught the simple basic skills of medicine and surgery. The term dressers probably originated with the first aid personnel in the British military hierarchy whose primary function was to dress wounds on the battlefield.

These men learned to function independently because the doctors simply couldn't see all of the many sick people who needed attention. By the time I arrived in Africa, a quarter of a century later, we had a number of dressers who were quite sophisticated in their medical skills and knowledge. Some of them had been trained specifically to work with leprosy patients. Their loving care and dedication made a significant impact on the wretched lives of people suffering from, and deformed by, this terrible disease.

During my first month in Tanganyika, Veda took me out for a visit to one of our clinics. We drove fifteen miles on the Wembere Plains in the Rift Valley before we reached the village in which the clinic was located. During the rainy season the roads to this community were impassable even with four-wheel drive vehicles. We were met by the two dressers, Abeli and Nalingigwa, the only medical staff of this isolated facility which served several thousand people. Each was about forty years of age, had the equivalence of a fifth grade education, a year of training at Kiomboi Hospital and several years experience. As I watched them in action, I was amazed at how effectively they diagnosed and treated a variety of illnesses. They had a microscope with which they identified malaria and parasitic disorders. Their pharmacy contained only a few simple drugs which these men knew how to use well and safely. Most frequently prescribed were quinine for malaria, aspirin for aches and pains, sulfa drugs for certain infections, and medication to eradicate worms. I believe that these two men were instrumental in curing as many people with serious illness and saving as many lives as the average family doctor back in America.

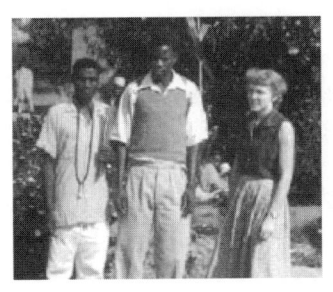

Veda with Iramba dressers

About the time we arrived in Tanganyika, the colonial medical services mandated that the training of personnel responsible for diagnosis and treatment be upgraded. Dressers were to be gradually replaced by medical assistants and doctors. This edict was something of a blow to the pride and prestige of some of our fine dressers who had diligently cared for their patients for years. Several of our dressers took additional training and became laboratory technicians at our hospitals.

One of these, Nikodemo, worked with me during my first year at Iambi Hospital. He was a warm and friendly man with a radiant smile, and accepted graciously the transition from taking personal care of patients to working in the laboratory. He became expert at diagnosing malaria with the microscope and doing skin smears for leprosy. We doctors learned to respect and appreciate his expertise and he became a vital member of our hospital team. He had a strong Christian faith and was constantly reaching out to see in what way he could help others. He made me smile and feel better about myself when I was down in the dumps.

Nikodemo had been retired for several years when we returned to Iambi in 1987. I was told that he was anxious to see us. We found him seated outside his modest cinder-block house with his wife. He recognized me immediately and arose to shake my hand and give me a big hug. Well into his seventies, Nikodemo appeared frail, his hair had become snow white, and his frame a little stooped, but he was just as alert and cheerful as ever. We spent a delightful half hour getting caught up on each other's lives. When it was time to say goodbye, he gently took my hand. With tears in his eyes he said, "Kweli tutaonana tena mbinguni!" (Surely we will meet again in heaven!) I must confess that my eyes weren't dry either. To me, Nikodemo and many other dressers like him were among the real heroes of the early phases of our medical work in Africa.

As medical work in Iramba-Turuland expanded it became clear that more nurses were needed. Our American missionary nurses were overwhelmed and unable to devote the loving care and individual attention to each patient, which had become second nature to them. The obvious solution was to train African nurses who would not face the language and cultural barriers which handicapped the expatriate nurses.

Other Lutheran mission groups and the colonial medical services agreed to cooperate in the development and operation of a school of nursing at Kiomboi. Students were recruited and selected from the mountainous regions of the north, from the coastal areas around Dar es Salaam, from the Southern Highlands, and from our own Iramba Plateau. The colonial medical services told us what should be taught but it was up to our missionary nursing staff to write lesson plans and provide necessary books and study materials.

Training African nurses challenged the ingenuity and patience of our American nursing faculty. The concept of married women working outside of their domestic duties at home was new and foreign. Partly for this reason it was decided to train young men as well as women. This led to some difficulty because the male students anticipated having a higher status than their female classmates.

Another major issue arose in getting students from different tribes to work together. We weren't far removed from the days of tribal warfare and some tribes still remembered old grievances. In that respect they weren't much different than Norwegian and Swedish immigrants to America a hundred years ago. Tribes from different corners of Tanganyika were culturally as different as urban New Yorkers and rural Texans. Many appeals had to be made for Christian understanding, love, and forgiveness with each new class of students. Fortunately, the American nurses who directed the Kiomboi Nurses Training School, Helen Erickson and Alice Turnbladh, were patient, caring individuals. They were able, by example, to teach the interaction and reconciliation necessary for students from different tribes to accept one another. They were ably assisted by all the other missionary nurses at Kiomboi including Jean Mykelbust, Margaret Peterson, Pauline Swanson, Martha Fosse, Greta Engberg, Freda Ohman, Veda Hult, Ann Saf, Elna Mae Lindahl, and others. Adeline was one of several missionary wives involved in teaching English to the nursing students while we were at Kiomboi.

The first class, made up of students who had graduated from the eighth grade, began their studies in 1953 and graduated in 1956. General education was still in its early stages of development in Tanganyika and this was the highest educational level of the students available for nurses' training. Some of those selected were only sixteen years of age. All of them were bright young men and women, having to be near the top of their classes in primary school to be picked for the limited number of openings in Middle School. From there competition for the few spaces in nurses' training was even more selective.

Some of the students came from families which were very poor and didn't even have money for shoes. During the first year of training, it was a quaint and charming experience to observe some of the students moving gracefully and silently around the hospital in their bare feet. The female students had been provided with attractive green pinstriped nurse's uniforms and the males with green shirts, white shorts and stockings. They all took pride in their physical appearance and cleanliness. The patients seemed pleased to be attended by such neat, handsome young nurses from their own land.

The faculty of KNTC literally performed miracles in turning out fine devoted nurses who served their people well. This was all the more amazing because their culture really had no counterpart to the devoted, unselfish Florence Nightingale tradition which is a part of our nursing heritage.

When it was mandated that all of our medical records be kept in English, we had some interesting and amusing applications of our American idioms recorded in our hospital records. One night a terminally man was admitted to the hospital. He was obviously dying. The student on duty recorded the following information on the official hospital chart:

"11:30 PM: Elderly gentleman admitted to men's ward with one foot in grave."

"12:00 PM: Other foot followed."

Another student nurse heard that I was making a trip to her home village on a day when she would be free from classes or hospital duty. She had obtained permission to visit her family for the day and asked me for a ride in the following manner, "Daktari, could you please jack me up at the nurses' dormitory at saa mbili (the second hour) tomorrow morning?" She had heard that when you had a flat tire you jacked up the vehicle and she logically concluded that when a passenger climbed into your car he or she was being jacked up, too.

She used the East African mode of indicating the time. The hours of the day and of the night are determined by sunrise and sunset. Near the equator the appearance and disappearance of the sun are always within minutes of six o'clock, twelve hours apart. Therefore saa mbili, the second hour, would be eight o'clock in the morning and saa mbili ya usiku would be eight o'clock at night.

We had many chuckles in working with our students from their ingenious and imaginative use of English, but we know that they had even more laughs from our bloopers as we stumbled through the Swahili language.

When Adeline and I revisited Irambaland thirty years later, we thoroughly enjoyed our reunion with the nurses we had helped train and with whom we had worked. One was the head nurse of the 400-bed Iambi Hospital. One lovely lady was the revered nurse-midwife of Iambi Hospital who had delivered thousands of babies over the years. Another was the wife of the doctor-in-charge of the hospital. Most of the women nurses were mothers and grandmothers, leaders and role models in their communities and churches. One had been elected to the national legislative body. One of our male nurses had gone to the seminary and become an ordained pastor. We were delighted to see and hear about all of their accomplishments, and gratified to know that we had played at least a small role in their development as good nurses and caring adults.

As the general educational level of Tanganyika rose, it became important to increase the sophistication of medical training. One route would have been to immediately establish medical schools comparable to those in America and Europe, but this would have been unrealistic, too time-consuming, and prohibitively expensive. The colonial and mission medical leaders felt that it would be much more appropriate to train a category of personnel known as medical assistants in relatively large numbers. They would be able to deliver basic health services under the supervision of government and mission doctors and nurses.

The Lutheran missions of Tanganyika banded together to establish a school to train medical assistants at Bumbuli in the northern mountainous region of the country. Applicants were to be male students who had successfully completed the Standard-10 examinations and showed maturity and an aptitude for dealing well with people. There was a great deal of competition for the openings for medical assistant training. I believe that most of the young men who were accepted would have been able to qualify as medical doctors in the USA if they had been afforded the appropriate educational opportunities.

The curriculum was set up to be completed in three years. The first year encompassed the basic sciences of anatomy, biochemistry, physiology, pathology, and pharmacology. The second two years were devoted to clinical training in which the students diagnosed and treated all of the common ailments prevalent in Africa. They also assisted the doctors and nurses in the operating room and learned to perform some basic surgical procedures.

Medical assistant students were not taught to deliver babies or deal specifically with gynecological problems because African women would be less willing to accept African men in these roles. Female students did not become medical assistants. They were to focus on nursing and midwifery.

From the time the school at Bumbuli opened, outstanding young men from Iramba-Turuland were recruited and sent for medical assistant training. Several of them had graduated and were at work at both Iambi and Kiomboi Hospitals when we arrived in 1957. Essentially they functioned as their communities' general practitioners, but often they had to assume full responsibility for staggering problems because no trained consultants were available. I was pleasantly surprised at the breadth of their knowledge and the caring wisdom with which they dealt with their patients.

Being a part of the culture and speaking the local languages fluently, they had an advantage over us American doctors. I found myself having to turn to them many times for help.

On the other hand, when they had made a diagnosis, they sometimes tended not to look further for other problems. Frequently our patients had multiple afflictions. For example, on one of my first days at Kiomboi Hospital an infant had been diagnosed as having the dreaded malady, cerebral malaria. The blood smear showed numerous malaria parasites under the microscope and the baby was nearly comatose. That added up to cerebral malaria, but when I examined the child I also noted a significant stiffness of the neck. I performed a spinal tap and found the fluid filled with pus cells and bacteria which clearly established the second diagnosis of meningitis. Death would have been almost certain without specific antibiotics. We treated the little girl intensively with penicillin and sulfa and she recovered completely. The medical assistant who admitted the baby never forgot that lesson.

The identical experience occurred later with two other babies but with different caregivers. I hasten to add that each of them had so many patients to see that it was almost inevitable that such oversights would occur. And I know that more than once I missed important diagnoses under similar circumstances.

One of the most eloquent tributes to our medical assistants has come from Dr. J. B. Dibble, an outstanding American surgeon who followed me at Kiomboi. He dedicated his book *This Land of Eve*, written about his African experiences, to Medical Assistant Sampson Paulo and to Mission Doctor Joe Norquist. Sampson died in 1964 of overwhelming hepatitis. Dr. Dibble's dedication reads:

"To Mr. Sampson Paulo, who was born in the African Bush, who died there in the springtime of his life, and who demonstrated with his life how well the African can be trained in the sciences."

I had worked with Sampson when he first came to our hospital and would add that he was one of the most dedicated, caring healers I have ever known.

After Tanganyika became independent in 1961, a medical school was established in Dar es Salaam. Many of the medical assistants returned to school and achieved their MD degrees. In 1987, most of the medical assistants with whom I had worked had gone to medical school and become doctors. Dr. Daudi Dyauli had been selected to be the doctor-in-charge of the expanded 400-bed Iambi Hospital. After medical school he had gone to Edinburgh, Scotland, for post-graduate training in pediatrics. He was a fine dedicated Christian who was a leader both at the hospital and at church. I was delighted to have him lead us on a tour of the new hospital at Iambi. We met colleagues with whom we had worked three decades earlier and even visited some patients who remembered me.

When we left Tanganyika in 1961 I had grown to care deeply for the Africans who had been my medical colleagues. The sadness of departure from the continent of my birth was eased somewhat by the knowledge that the work which we had done was being carried on by the medical personnel with whom we had worked during their formative years.

10. A DAY OF GREAT SORROW

Our African friends in Iramba-Turuland were intimately familiar with the loss of loved ones, both among the very young and at any age thereafter. For our first three months in Tanganyika we were full-time Swahili language students. I was only to be called to the hospital twenty-five miles away for emergencies. The first five patients I was summoned to examine and treat all died! By the time I saw them, there was nothing I could do to save any one of them. This was a horrendous experience for an American pediatrician new to the pervasiveness of death in this awakening continent. I grieved with the bereaved families and had difficulty sleeping at night.

The father of a young man who had just died of a ruptured appendix was surprised at the intensity of my emotional involvement. I declared that we could probably have saved his son if we had seen him earlier. The elderly gentleman was obviously grief-stricken, but he gently comforted me. He said, "But Daktari, don't you understand that this was the will of God, and you couldn't have done anything that would have changed it!" I started to counter his statement, but realized that nothing I could say about such fatalism would be of solace or comfort to him.

Familiarity with death does not mute the pangs of grief. The bereft African relatives and friends suffered their losses intensely and for many days. On one occasion a baby died in her mother's arms just as she reached Iambi Hospital. The grieving parent was informed that the doctor was in the operating room. She charged in and laid her infant on the open abdomen of the patient who was having surgery, seriously complicating the operation being performed. In anguished cries, she implored the doctor to save her baby, but there was nothing he could do.

When death involved our African coworkers or their families, we missionaries shared their sorrows. The death of a lovely young African friend which most painfully affected me occurred at Iambi Hospital in 1957.

Daudi Dyauli had become special to me both as a colleague and as a friend. Before we arrived in Tanganyika, our missionary medical staff had watched with interest and excitement the romance which developed between Daudi and Salome, one of the first graduates of the Kiomboi Nurses Training School. She was the granddaughter of Mama Salome, the wonderful midwife who had given years of dedicated service to our medical work. Salome was a delightful young woman and a fine nurse. Everybody agreed that she and David were made for each other. Much joy and excitement attended the announcement of their engagement, and their wedding was celebrated happily by their relatives, the African church, and the mission family.

David and Salome were settled in their first home at Iambi when we arrived. I was excited when they came to me with the news that Salome was pregnant and honored when they asked me to deliver the baby. The young mother-to-be took good care of herself and the pregnancy proceeded normally. Her pelvic measurements seemed adequate and all other findings indicated that she should have a normal delivery. I looked forward to participating in the arrival of a much-wanted and prayed-for addition to the family of Salome and David!

Labor began one evening soon after sunset. Both of our missionary nurses, Amy Larson and Alpha Jacques, were close at hand throughout the night. Another experienced nurse, Helen Pedersen, was available to administer anesthesia if necessary. Strong contractions continued through the night, and I examined Salome regularly. As the painful hours passed, she remained brave and composed, but she was visibly becoming more tired and anxious. The mouth of her uterus was opening slowly but the baby's head was too large to descend into the pelvis. After twelve hours of hard labor there was virtually no progress. Then the infant's heart rate began to slow alarmingly and Salome's blood pressure dropped enough for us to be concerned about impending shock. The baby's head was too high for a safe forceps delivery so the only solution was a Caesarean section.

We discussed the urgent situation with Salome and David. They agreed that we should go ahead with the operation. Preparations were made as rapidly as possible and Salome was taken into the operating room. Before anesthesia, one of our nurses prayed fervently in Swahili for the welfare of mother and child. I made the incision through the lower abdominal wall, opened the uterus and lifted out a chubby little girl. As I aspirated her nose and mouth with a syringe she vigorously protested with a lusty cry. I could hear David's happy laugh outside the operating room as he heard this new exciting sound and was told that he had a beautiful daughter. During the delivery of the placenta, the nurse administering anesthesia reported that the blood pressure was dropping rapidly. We hurried the closure of the incisions, but the blood pressure continued falling. In spite of our efforts, Salome quickly descended into deep shock and her heart stopped. All of our efforts to resuscitate her were unsuccessful. The previous aura of joy at the baby's arrival was transformed into overwhelming sadness. These moments were comparable to the most horrible bad dream I had ever experienced. I just prayed that I would awaken and find out that it wasn't so, that Salome would open her eyes and ask to see her daughter. All of us in the operating room were in emotional shock. I am not exaggerating when I state that for me this was the saddest, most crushing moment of my entire career as a physician.

David, waiting outside, could sense that something was badly amiss. After I realized that there was no hope for reviving Salome and saw that the baby was fine, I slipped off my surgical mask and stepped out. David was standing with members of his and Salome's family. When I told him the news he was devastated and was immediately surrounded and consoled by his loved ones. I was speechless and stepped away, leaving them to their collective grieving.

I was so overwhelmed that I had to get away by myself. A hundred yards behind the hospital stood a beautiful candelabra (euphorbia) tree next to a giant termite mound. Between them I had discovered a nook where I could sit on a projection of the ant hill and be completely concealed from all but one direction. On a couple of happier occasions, I had escaped to this refuge for moments of solitude and meditation. On this fateful day I hurried to my special hiding place, sat down with my face in my hands and simply wept for several minutes.

"Why had I become a doctor?"

"What was I doing here in Africa?"

"Why did this beautiful young mother have to die?"

"Why hadn't I recognized the seriousness of the problem earlier?"

"Why didn't we have blood available to treat the shock?"

"Why hadn't I taken more training in obstetrical emergencies?" (I had delivered over 150 babies but was woefully inexperienced in dealing with childbirth emergencies because I had always had consultants available.)

"Would David, Salome's mother, and her family forgive me; and how would he cope?"

"What would be the future of this darling little girl who had lost her mother?"

I have no idea how long I grieved alone before I heard a kindly voice calling me. Rev. Ruben Pedersen, president of our Iramba-Turu mission, was at that time stationed at Iambi. His wife Helen, who had given the anesthesia, called him to the hospital immediately after Salome's death. He came looking for me and soon discovered my sanctuary. This kind friend and pastor gently urged me to consider how much I was needed as the only doctor at Iambi. He was no stranger to grief himself, having lost his first wife to illness in Africa. He helped me put things in perspective by his counsel and a prayer for comfort and healing. Then he urged me to go home and share my sorrow with Adeline. This I did, and she was able to help me immensely with her understanding, comfort and love. Adeline herself was seven months pregnant, so this tragedy held relevant emotional implications for us.

David's grief was deep but he continued his excellent work at the hospital. He named his daughter Salome after her mother. With the help of his family, she thrived in every respect. After an appropriate time, David courted and married Eliwaza, one of Salome's nursing school classmates.

During our visit in 1987, Eliwaza confided that Salome had had a premonition that she might not survive the labor and delivery. If she died, she hoped that Eliwaza would marry David and become the mother of her baby. Eliwaza was not only a fine nurse but became an effective leader of the women's work of the church. She and David had several children, two of whom were at home. We were not able to meet Salome because she was teaching in Dar es Salaam.

Forty years have passed but Salome's death remains a vivid and terribly painful memory. Yet through this tragedy, I have learned much about the special dimensions of grief and love, and ultimate healing. These lessons have been especially meaningful to me as a physician and as a human being.

11. "YOU TEACH ME YOUR MEDICINE AND I'LL TEACH YOU MINE!"

One morning while examining a patient in my office, I was startled by noisy activity in the hall outside. I heard a knock on the door and an urgent voice calling, "Daktari, we need you!" Responding immediately, I was confronted by a dramatic scene. An excited group surrounded the bed which they had carried into the hallway. On it lay an emaciated middle-aged man who was coughing up blood. He was conscious and alert but visibly frightened.

Ntindilo was introduced to me as an Iramba medicine man from a village about thirty miles from Kiomboi. Over the past few months, his chronic cough had become worse with fever and much weight loss. He had been treating himself with many different herbal medicines to no avail. After he began to cough up increasing amounts of blood, he asked the members of his clan to take him to Kiomboi Hospital.

He appeared seriously ill with an elevated temperature and a rapid heart rate. With my stethoscope I heard distinct abnormalities in both lungs. We needed an x-ray. Our small U.S. Army surplus unit was powered by an ancient and temperamental gasoline generator. Our staff hadn't been trained to use this equipment, so it was up to me to get the machine going. I cranked long and hard, saying a few bad words under my breath, with no results. I checked the spark plug, adjusted the choke lever, and tried again. Finally, the old engine reluctantly sputtered to life. We carefully placed our patient in position and I took x-rays of his chest. Then I discovered that our developing solutions were outdated. Replacing them and processing the film consumed at least an hour. At last we had our pictures which showed typical findings of advanced tuberculosis with large cavities in both lungs.

Ntindilo was admitted to our small isolation unit which was set apart from the rest of the hospital. One of his family stayed with him to prepare his meals. We started treating him with three anti-tuberculosis drugs, INH, PAS, and streptomycin. I was concerned that our treatment wouldn't be effective at this advanced stage of his disease. During the first two weeks of his hospital care, there was no apparent improvement. He was listless and apathetic with very little interest in his surroundings. Gradually his fever came down, his appetite returned, and he became more alert.

Over the next few weeks there was a dramatic transformation in our patient. When we made rounds, he welcomed us with a contagious grin. He asked relevant questions about everything we did. My stethoscope fascinated him. He apparently believed that it was inhabited by powerful spirits. If I was slow to listen to his chest, he would remind me by pointing to the stethoscope and then to his heart. He was absolutely dumbfounded when I showed him his chest x-ray. I indicated the outlines of his heart and his lungs with the plainly visible holes in them. He declared that the machine must have powerful spirits to look inside him like that.

He soon made friends with everybody on our staff. He was particularly fond of our young blonde American head nurse, Jean Mykelbust. She was a warm, outgoing person who radiated care and concern for each patient. One day when she and I came into his room he declared, "Both of you have become special to me. I like to think of you, Bibi Jean, as my mother; and I like to think of you, Daktari, as my son!" She was a bit taken aback. Although she was a motherly person, he was old enough to be her father. Perhaps he was confused about her chronological age because Africans had difficulty distinguishing between blond and gray hair. Blondes seemed to be accorded more respect than brunettes. On the other hand, it may have been just a figurative declaration of affection and appreciation. Jean and I both accepted his claim on us as a special compliment.

Ntindilo was by nature an inveterate tease. One day he called attention to my ponderous gait, saying, "You walk like an elephant!" I noticed that he was grinning as he spoke. Other Africans had said the same thing about my stride which had probably originated from my days of walking behind a horse-drawn plow many years earlier. In response I sought every opportunity to get back at Ntindilo. For some time he had been asking me to remove a half-inch mole on his lower leg. When we finally had some free time in the operating room, I said to him, "Okay, we'll take that thing off tomorrow." In preparation I asked the nurse to sterilize the necessary instruments. Then I requested that she add three wicked-looking tools to the instrument pack: a large bone chisel, a heavy stainless steel hammer, and a gleaming amputation saw.

Next morning, with a trusting smile, my patient climbed on the operating table. I injected the mole with Novocain and began placing the instruments on the tray. Using a sterile forceps, I lifted each implement out so he could see it. When I got to the chisel and hammer his eyes widened. As the amputation saw came into view, he yelped, jumped off the table, and fled out of the room. When I finally caught up with him, it took considerable persuasion to satisfy him that I wasn't really going to use those lethal weapons. I was just pulling his leg but he was afraid that I was going to saw it off. Eventually we got him back to the operating room and removed his mole. He wanted to keep the surgical specimen. Perhaps he thought that if I kept that little piece of his body its spirit might come back to haunt him.

One day he made a startling proposition. He looked me straight in the eye and said, "If you will teach me your medicine, I will teach you mine!" I explained that our knowledge was stored in books which we western doctors referred to every day. His proposition would be impossible unless he learned to read. His response was, "Well then, teach me!" We accepted that challenge. A student nurse volunteered to help. Using adult literacy materials and a Swahili primer, the volunteer teacher put him to work. Each day when we arrived for rounds, he was busy with his books and asked many questions. Within a month he proudly demonstrated that we could pick out any page in his primary school reader and he would zip through it. He also practiced writing and made good progress.

Then came the morning when we found him very depressed. All his books and writing material had disappeared. When I asked him about it, he said, "It's no use! And besides, I can make more money than you any day! All you charge is a few shillings. When I treat a patient I get a cow!" He had reached the conclusion that the obstacles to becoming a new type of doctor were too formidable. I felt guilty that I hadn't made that clear to him from the start. I did point out to him that his developing reading skill could still greatly enrich his life. Later we did catch him studying on his own.

What did I learn from Ntindilo? Our time was so limited and our cultural gap so great that I couldn't really enter his world. I did learn to appreciate and respect him. He was a man who really cared for his people, a true healer. I'm certain that he helped many by using only the methods he had learned in a long apprenticeship. He functioned in a world of powerful spirits and used all his powers to get them to release their hold on his patients. He even practiced a form of preventive medicine: some patients paid him to keep them well. He was reluctant to discuss certain aspects of his practice. For one thing the practice of native medicine had been outlawed by the government.

Another medicine man had come to me earlier and asked if we could go into business together. By putting his medicines into the empty capsules we had in our pharmacy, he assumed that they would become legitimate. We could make a killing! Of course I had to veto that proposition.

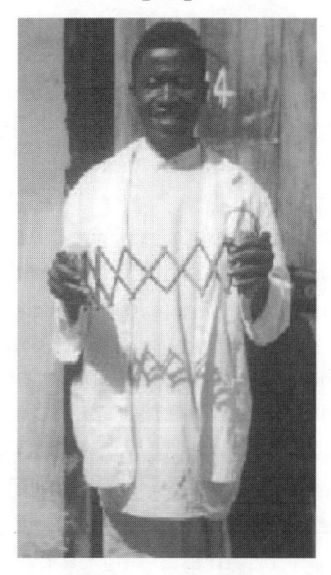

Ntindilo, wearing my white coat, with a diagnostic tool.

African medicine men did indeed have some potent medicines which could kill worms, purge the bowels, stimulate the heart, and relieve the pain. On the other hand, there was no concept of dosage. I saw a number of patients die from the effects of native medicine. Most of them became jaundiced with total liver failure. Never did the families blame the Mgangas. People died because they were bewitched or it was just "Shauri la Mungu"(the will of God).

After a year at our hospital, Ntindilo's tuberculosis was arrested. He had gained twenty pounds and felt better than he had for years. X-rays showed damaged lung tissue which would have been best removed surgically. In Tanganyika in 1960 that was not feasible. A few weeks before discharge, he begged me to give him one of my old white coats. At first I hesitated and then relented. "What harm can it possibly do?" The day came for him to go home. In parting he said, "Kwa Heri!" and gently shook my hand. (Africans don't go for bone-crushing handshakes.) My eyes were moist as I watched him walk slowly into the African bush wearing my old white coat.

12. "AN EYE FOR AN EYE; AND A NOSE FOR A NOSE!"

I am not a surgeon! My three years in postgraduate pediatric training, two years as an Army medical officer, and two years of general practice had not prepared me for all the surgical challenges which I would encounter in Tanganyika. Thousands of patients needed surgery but no surgeons practiced in our area. Frequently, an emergency operation held the only possibility of saving a life. On many other occasions, wielding the scalpel was vital to restoring useful function. In the absence of fully trained surgeons, we medical missionaries on the front line felt obliged to do the best we could to save lives and correct major problems. More often than not, the results were satisfying and appreciated. We occasionally experienced frustration and failure.

One day a young man was carried to the hospital in great distress. Both sides of his lower jaw were broken causing it to be angled far to the right. Although it was painfully difficult to talk, he was able to explain that he had been walking home at night and fallen into a deep gully. I suspected that it was more likely that his chin had had a violent collision with another man's fist or club. At any rate, he needed help. I had never treated such a fracture before but knew that one effective procedure consisted in wiring the upper and lower jaw teeth together. With the bones held securely, the fractures could heal.

We sedated the patient, injected local anesthesia, and I straightened out the ugly deformity. Since I had neither the proper equipment nor the experience, it took more than two hours to fix the wires around the upper and lower molars and fasten them together. When I was finished, the jaw looked perfectly straight and was snugly immobilized. In those days the Iramba adults filed off the inner corners of the central incisor teeth as a form of tribal identification. This gave our patient a nice gap through which he could take liquids and soft food.

I was delighted and highly satisfied with my morning's work. When I went home for lunch, I told Adeline that I had finally done something in the operating room which looked just like the picture in the textbook. Now all we had to do was keep our patient quiet and teach him to take his nourishment through the gap between his front teeth. Our nurses patiently showed him how he could eat uji, a thin porridge cooked from ground millet. He did this easily and was able to take other soft and pureed foods. Drinking liquids was no problem at all.

After three days in the hospital, he insisted on going home. We carefully explained to him that his jaw had to remain wired shut for at least six weeks. He assured me that he understood and would return to see me in ten days.

When he returned on the appointed day, I was horrified to see that his mouth was open and his broken jaw angled off to the right even worse than before I had patched him up. All of our work had been in vain! He explained that after a week his jaw felt fine; he was sure that it was healed. The wires became so uncomfortable that with great effort he took them off. He wouldn't have come back to see me but there was one wire that he just couldn't get off. I was so upset that I told him he could just keep that little strand of metal around his tooth to remember me by. I never saw him again but often imagined him, with his lop-sided jaw, telling his grandchildren about that strange white doctor who wired his mouth shut.

Later at Kiomboi Hospital, a woman came in with her face covered. In a fit of anger her husband had bitten off the end of her nose. The missing part had not been recovered. My colleague, Dr. Dennis Lofstrom, who had had some experience in plastic surgery, confidently declared, "Let's make her a new nose!" I assisted him as he prepared a one-inch tube of skin from the inside of her left forearm. With her wrist against her forehead and her fingers resting on the top of her head, he sewed the end of the flap to the remainder of the nose. The other end was still part of the forearm and provided the blood supply. We then applied a plaster cast around the head, hand, and upper arm to securely hold everything together. This was to remain in place for two weeks. I marveled at how patiently she endured this miserably uncomfortable ordeal.

Fourteen days later the skin from the forearm had grown to the nose. We removed the cast and Denny severed the flap leaving one end attached to the nose. This he carefully sewed in place so that she indeed did have a new nose which didn't look too bad. After gravely inspecting her new face in the mirror, our patient smiled. A day later she was discharged.

On the very next day, a man came to the clinic missing the end of his nose. Although we hadn't anticipated such a chain reaction, we weren't totally surprised with the news that he was the husband of Lady New-nose. She had extracted her revenge. Now he figured that Dr. Lofstrom could fix him, too, and perhaps even improve on the original model. We accordingly went through the initial steps and bound him up with an extra sturdy cast to hold his forearm to his nose. But, alas! He wasn't as patient and long-suffering as his wife. By the next morning he had broken the cast and torn his arm loose. He decided that it was better to live without a nose than to go through that ordeal.

Such domestic tragedies aren't confined to Africa. When I was a medical student in St. Louis I helped take care of a man whose wife had bitten off his ear, apparently for good reasons.

Not all of my adventures in surgery ended in frustration. One of the most gratifying experiences of my medical career occurred during our first weeks in Africa. We were assigned to the Isanzu Mission Station for six weeks of Swahili language study with Bob and Jeanne Ward as our hosts. The nearest hospital was twenty-five miles away but Isanzu had a fairly well-equipped dispensary. I wasn't supposed to be seeing patients while devoting my efforts to learning our new language, but exceptions were made for emergencies or special cases. One day I was called to the clinic after a pleasant young man named Abeli had walked in with his wife from their home at least ten miles away. His wife Raheli was a tall graceful woman in her early twenties nursing a chubby alert six-month-old baby. As we were being introduced, she was covering her face with her left hand. Initially I thought this was a gesture of shyness and modesty. I was captivated by Raheli's beautiful brown eyes, but sensed in her gaze a definite sadness. As I admired her baby, Abeli volunteered the information that this was their daughter and that they had two older children at home.

When Raheli removed her hand from her face, I was startled to see that her beauty was marred by a grotesque hare lip. The upper lip was completely cleft near the mid-line with the ends sagging down over her teeth. As a result, her nostrils were uneven and greatly distorted. Abeli politely asked if we could help her.

My initial reaction was skeptical. I was not a plastic surgeon and we had only primitive equipment. There wasn't even the remotest possibility that she could get to a larger medical center so I thought, "I can at least try!" I had assisted a surgeon in Minneapolis while he repaired cleft lips and could see what needed to be done.

I thought of the ordeals through which this pleasant young woman must have lived. In the first place, her mother must have been patient and loving to overcome the difficulties of breast feeding her baby with no functioning upper lip. Then there was the stigma of her deformity which can be devastating in any society. I looked at the imploring eyes of the husband who obviously adored her. I told them that we would try to fix her lip and it could be done right away. My medical bag contained a small sterile surgical pack with the necessary instruments.

Raheli reclined on the examining table and we prepared her face with antiseptic solution. Using Novocain anesthesia, I trimmed the edges of the gaping lip and carefully sewed them together. I was pleasantly surprised at how the edges fit together. Fortunately, the front teeth were quite regular and the palate was intact so there was no speech disorder. I applied a snug supportive dressing and asked her to return in three days.

Raheli stayed with a relative who lived near the clinic and came in twice for dressing changes. On the tenth day I removed the bandage and the stitches. She had become a beautiful woman! I'll never forget her look of delight when she first beheld her new face in a mirror. Abeli also was beaming with joy and pride. He had loved her simply for who she was for a long time. Now her physical loveliness became apparent for all to see. I was deeply moved, and felt uniquely privileged to have been a participant.

13. POLIO COMES TO IAMBI

I spent the first year in Africa working at our fifty-bed hospital at Iambi. There I had my initial experience with polio in the tropics. In 1949 while serving my internship at St. Louis City Hospital, our staff had been overwhelmed by a devastating polio epidemic. All of our available beds were filled with acute paralytic cases. Four iron-lung respirators were constantly in use. Over one 24-hour period three of us interns performed over one hundred spinal taps on suspected cases. Fourteen of these patients were admitted to the hospital with paralysis or other complications. Most of the milder cases were sent home after the spinal fluid examination ruled out meningitis. Many of those afflicted were adolescents and young adults. When our first case appeared at Iambi eight years later, I shuddered, expecting to go through the same nightmare again.

In America a century ago, the disease was called infantile paralysis because it primarily attacked babies and small children. Over the years it began affecting older children and young adults. Improved sanitation and higher hygienic standards impeded the spread of the virus through the population until a virulent epidemic came along.

Polio in Africa presented an entirely different face. In developing countries there is more frequent presence of the virus in intestinal secretions. A pioneer study in Egypt indicated that most babies had protective polio antibodies by the time they were a year old. They were exposed at a time when they had some "transient" immunity from their mothers resulting in mild non-paralytic polio which gave lifelong protection. At Iambi we did not see a single child over three with paralysis and most of the afflicted babies were less severely ill than those we had cared for in St. Louis. There was one dramatic and tragic exception.

Martin Luther Gunda was a beautiful bright-eyed fifteen-month-old child. His father Zephania, who had earlier been a well-liked teacher and school administrator, was one of the first Iramba pastors to graduate from our seminary in northern Tanganyika. He was an effervescent, happy extrovert who related well to everybody around him. His deep Christian faith was obvious. In 1957 he was sent to Minneapolis for further theological training.

Martin's mother Wanzelia was a warm radiant person whom we all loved. Since the birth of her only child Samuel five years earlier, her health had been fragile. An additional sadness came into their lives when the Gundas discovered that Samuel was legally blind. Wanzelia and Zephania despaired of having any more children, so when she became pregnant, they were delighted. After a difficult nine months, a healthy baby boy joined the family. The parents and big brother were ecstatic and the new arrival was considered to be a miracle baby, an answer to their prayers. It had already been decided that he was to be named Martini Luteri.

From birth this little boy was the focal point of a happy close-knit family. He was distinctly precocious, walking alone well before his first birthday. Even more remarkable was his language development. By one year he combined words into sentences. And he loved music. He could carry a tune and sing all the words to one of the African children's hymns, Mungu Ni Pendo (God Is Love). Our children, Margaret, Elly and Dan, were fond of him.

Only two weeks after his father had flown to America, little Martin developed a high fever. Wanzelia brought him to the hospital where we immediately recognized that he was seriously ill. The malaria smear was negative. His neck was stiff and he was clearly having difficulty breathing. He was unable to swallow the saliva accumulating in his throat. After doing a spinal tap, we found that he had an increase in the type of white blood cells in the spinal fluid which predominate in polio. When he cried, his voice had a nasal quality and he had weakness of the respiratory and swallowing muscles. He had severe bulbar polio and should have been put in a respirator, but we had no such equipment at Iambi. All we could do was give an ineffective type of artificial respiration and repeatedly suction the saliva from his mouth and throat.

As each hour passed, his respiratory efforts became weaker, his fever higher, and his color more blue. His feeble cry was heart-rending. Gradually he lapsed into unconsciousness and died within twenty-four hours. We were all stunned! Our two American nurses and all the African staff wept openly. Through her tears Wanzelia maintained a serene Madonna-like composure. She was more worried about the shock of the news upon her husband in Minneapolis than she was concerned about herself.

In Tanganyika a funeral was conducted by sunset on the day of the death. Most of the family lived in the vicinity of Iambi. Late in the afternoon, they were joined in the church by a host of friends and all the missionary family who were able to attend. The service was conducted by our Iramba pastor, Rev. Simeon Petro. The plain tiny casket was carried to the nearby cemetery with the family following closely. After the burial the family remained at the graveside, singing hymns until late in the evening. They were lead by the clear sweet voice of the grieving mother Wanzelia. The contrast between this serene, hope-filled funeral and the anguished, wailing of a pagan death dance projected a powerful message to all of us.

Our children were deeply affected by little Martin Luther's death. This was their first experience with the loss of a child whom they had known and cared for. They asked many poignant questions.

We had only three more cases of toddlers with paralytic polio at Iambi after Martin's death. They all recovered with only slight leg muscle weakness. For every case with paralysis, there were probably hundreds with mild infections which resulted in lifetime immunity.

We were concerned about our own children who had received the brand new Salk vaccine just before we left for Africa. I still wasn't convinced of its effectiveness. We did not have access to the oral vaccine in Tanganyika and our three did not receive it until we returned to America in 1961.

Two years after Martin's death, I attended a World Health Organization conference in Kampala, Uganda. One of the speakers, Dr. Omonde, gave a dramatic account of their trial of the new Sabin oral vaccine in an epidemic raging through a heavily populated district in Kenya. Over thirty new cases of paralytic polio were occurring per week. A public health team targeted the center of the outbreak. Over a five-day period they sprayed the vaccine into the mouths of over 60,000 children. The campaign was too late to protect the twenty new cases which developed that week. The next week there were only five new cases and this dropped to one the following seven-day period. After the third week no further paralytic cases occurred. The epidemic had been stopped in its tracks!

Dr. Omonde's voice trembled with emotion as he finished his presentation.

In 1956 while studying tropical medicine at Tulane University, I had heard Dr. Albert Sabin lecture about his new vaccine. He was convinced that it was the most effective public health measure to control worldwide polio. Russia and several other European nations were already using it. Because there were still concerns about its safety, and because of the demonstration that the injected Salk killed-vaccine was both effective and safe, Dr. Sabin's vaccine had not been licensed in the United States.

We are still concerned about the universal use of oral polio vaccine. A tiny fraction of those receiving the oral form, about one in four million, can develop paralysis. Non-immune parents have been paralyzed when they picked up the vaccine virus from their recently immunized babies. This has resulted in multi-million-dollar lawsuits and a question about switching back to injected killed vaccines. However, the Sabin vaccine has been used effectively throughout the world and there is great hope among public health experts that soon after the turn of the century, polio will be totally eradicated. It would then join smallpox as a scourge no longer devastating mankind.

For little Martin Luther Gunda these protective measures came far too late!

14. FEVER OF THE MOSQUITO

Homa ya mbu translates into fever of the mosquito. Throughout human history, malaria has plagued mankind, primarily in the tropics and subtropics. In 1952 authorities estimated that 350 million cases occurred in the world annually, with an average mortality rate of one per cent. The greatest number of these 3.5 million deaths was suffered by infants, small children, and adults being infected for the first time.

Malaria is transmitted from person to person by Anopheles mosquitoes. A female mosquito picks up the male and female reproductive cells of the malaria parasite in its blood meal. These unite and develop into thousands of infective offspring in the body of the insect. When the mosquito bites another human, these new parasites invade the bloodstream and set up housekeeping in the liver. Here they multiply and develop into another stage which enters red blood cells, dividing repeatedly until the cell ruptures, releasing the enclosed parasites which attack the next set of blood cells. After an incubation period of ten to thirty days, the infected person experiences cycles of fever, headaches and chills every two to three days. These coincide with the simultaneous rupture of billions of red cells which had been invaded at the same time by the preceding generation of parasites. The cycles continue, getting worse until the patient is treated, the immune system responds, or death ensues.

In Irambaland we experienced malaria throughout the year. A sharp increase in the number of cases occurred during the rainy season, coinciding with the dramatic rise in the population of mosquitoes. Our clinics were busiest at this time of year with hundreds of people coming in daily for treatment of malaria. Almost every day we saw infants with the dreaded complication of cerebral malaria in which the small blood vessels of the brain are plugged by parasite-laden red cells. Many of these babies died before medication could take effect, and others expired before they could receive medical treatment.

We Americans, having no immunity from previous attacks, were highly vulnerable to malaria. One hundred years ago this disease was prevalent in our Southern States and along the

East Coast as far north as Boston. As a child in the Ozarks I remember hearing about doctors treating the neighbors for malaria. Our public health services virtually eliminated malaria through mosquito control, screened windows and medication with quinine. However, in rural Tanganyika, none of these methods could be effectively applied to the African population. Resources were simply too limited.

We expatriates took prophylactic medication, slept under mosquito nets, had screened windows, and tried to avoid outside exposure at night when malaria-bearing mosquitoes are active. Unfortunately, our initial preventive medication, paludrine, was not effective against the local strains of malaria. We took it faithfully every morning, but all six of our family had attacks during our first two years in Africa.

I was the first one to succumb. Edith Kjellin, one of our missionary nurses, an African dresser, and I were out on safari making dispensary visits. An hour after sundown our Jeep engine sputtered and died on a seldom traveled dirt road ten miles from the nearest settlement. Using every trick available, we tried unsuccessfully to get it started.

I had been feeling ill all afternoon and gradually developed a severe headache and violent shaking chills. Our dresser offered to set out for help but seemed relieved when we vetoed that suggestion. The surrounding countryside was populated by both lions and leopards. We decided to wait for assistance and settled in the vehicle for the night. As my symptoms increased, Edith was convinced that I had malaria. She insisted that I take the initial treatment dose of chloroquine. Although nauseated, I somehow managed to keep the pills down but kept getting worse. That night became one of the longest and most miserable in my life. I felt sorry for my companions because they seemed so anxious about my condition. The first light of dawn was brightening the eastern sky before anxious friends came to rescue us. By then I was feeling better and recovered rapidly.

My next attack, which was much more severe, hit me the day before we were scheduled to take Adeline from Iambi to Kiomboi to await the delivery of our little one. My headache was excruciating and my fever kept rising. I remember vividly the terrible pain in my eyeballs, teeth, back, and abdomen. There wasn't any part of me that didn't hurt. My body shook violently with chills at the same moment that my temperature was approaching 105 degrees Fahrenheit. Nausea and vomiting made it impossible to keep down my medication. It is said that with severe malaria one feels so sick that he's afraid that he is going to die. Then he gets worse and feels so bad that he fears that he won't die. That's exactly how my sentiments progressed during the attack.

Since no other doctors were around, Adeline sent for our friend Medical Assistant Daudi Dyauli. He started intravenous fluids containing a generous dose of choloroquine. I barely remember his presence but know that his prompt treatment may have saved my life. At the same time, Adeline had a positive smear and was taking choloroquine which made her nervous and depressed. By the next morning my fever had subsided and I was feeling a bit better.

Stan Alderson from the leprosarium drove us the fifty miles from Iambi to Kiomboi. That jolting ride seemed to go on forever, but we finally arrived. Adeline, who was having a few contractions, was settled into a room in our missionary 'Sick Bay.' Dr. Viola Fisher insisted that I be admitted to the adjoining room.

When Adeline's labor began, I was vaguely aware of its progression but too ill to actively participate. Martha, born with a forceps delivery, announced her presence with a lusty cry. I crawled out of bed to get my first glimpse of our healthy blond daughter but our nurses soon put me back in the prone position. The joy of this new addition to our family hastened my recovery.

During our first two years in Tanganyika, Adeline, Margaret, Elly, Dan and Martha all became ill with malaria. All four children had their first attacks during one terrible week in February of 1958. They probably had been infected a month earlier when we were stuck in a flooded river late at night. Each had a tummy ache so severe that we even worried about appendicitis in addition to the malaria. We had some anxious moments and little sleep until the children improved. Fourteen years earlier my father had died of complications of malaria in Dar es salaam. I couldn't help but remember, too, the little African patients I had lost recently to *homa ya mbu*. We were relieved and grateful when the children responded to treatment with choloroquine.

Because of numerous failures of paludrine prophylaxis, we doctors decided to try another approach. We settled on a preventive dose of chloroquine, to be taken once or twice weekly. Thereafter, we had no more malaria in our family. Our children hated chloroquine because of its terribly bitter taste, but they soon learned to put it on the back of the tongue and gulp it down quickly with water.

Several of the malaria drugs have frightening side effects. One of our adolescent African students became violently psychotic after being treated with atabrine. It took several strong men to restrain him until I could sedate him by injection. A mission doctor became so disoriented after taking camoquine that he didn't know who or where he was for two days. While taking chloroquine twice a week, Dan began having nightmares. One night he awoke screaming that there were ten thousand snakes in his room. On another occasion there were leopards outside his window. I convinced him that it was only a bad dream by taking him out the next morning and showing him that there were no tracks in the soft dust outside the house. Dr. Moris suggested that chloroquine might be involved and we determined that the bad nights had each followed the day he had taken his pill. We solved the problem by dividing the recommended amount of chloroquine into small doses given daily. Bingo! No more nightmares. Each time I took the full treatment dose of chloroquine I became quite depressed for several days. Many of my patients had the same experience.

We were informed in 1987 that malaria continued its devastation. Several strains of chloroquine-resistant malaria have appeared. The increased population density provides more people for each infected mosquito to bite. Financial resources are so meager that effective mosquito control and preventive medication are virtually impossible. As long as this is so, malaria will remain a major health problem in the Third World.

15. OUR YELLOW CHRISTMAS

On November 27, 1959, a special Thanksgiving feast was served at our boarding school for missionary children at Kiomboi. Most of the children lived too far away to go home for that holiday weekend. A total of seventy-eight children and adults from North America, Great Britain, Switzerland, and Scandinavia celebrated in the colorfully decorated school cafeteria. Some of the parents and guests had traveled several hours to be on hand and we were all enjoying the company of those we hadn't seen for many weeks. The children presented a brief program which highlighted the meaning of Thanksgiving.

Since turkeys weren't available in Tanganyika, our feast featured baked chicken with all the trimmings, including pumpkin pie. We especially enjoyed the delicious fruit salad containing papaya, mangoes, bananas, and pineapple. All of these came from our own Kiomboi shamba (orchard or garden). We agreed that the feast was almost as good as Thanksgiving at Grandma's house.

About three weeks later, several of the celebrants of the big feast became ill with fever, loss of appetite, dark urine, yellow skin, nausea, and vomiting. I became one of the first victims. One of our children exclaimed to me, "Daddy, your eyes are yellow!" By then, we knew that we were afflicted by some type of hepatitis. I felt awful and went to bed because I was too weak to stand up for more than a few minutes. Margaret and Elly soon developed the same symptoms, so Adeline had three bedfast patients on her hands. Over the next few weeks more than half of those eating that fateful meal developed the same symptoms, some much sicker than others.

A little detective work established that all of the yellow victims had attended our Kiomboi Thanksgiving and had eaten the fruit salad which had been prepared by one of the Iramba cooks who said that he had not been sick. One of our doctors examined him and found that he had a slightly enlarged tender liver and a discernible yellowing of the whites of his eyes. Since he had a mild case of hepatitis, he was the probable source of our outbreak. There was no way the school staff could have foreseen or prevented the food contamination.

The sequence of events suggested that our epidemic was caused by Type A hepatitis virus. Since the disease caused by this microorganism can be prevented or modified by gamma globulin shots, we immediately telegraphed an order to a South African pharmaceutical company. It was flown to Dar es Salaam and forwarded inland by rail and mail truck, arriving at Kiomboi ten days later. Injections were given to all the Americans and Europeans who had been exposed. This included Adeline, Dan, and Martha. The children weren't particularly enthused or appreciative. They wondered why they had to have a shot when they weren't sick.

We saw no new cases among the African population, including those who had eaten the fruit salad, so we did not give them gamma globulin. Apparently this virus was widely prevalent in our area and most local residents had developed immunity at an early age.

Margaret, Elly, and I were sickest on December 25th. In the tropics we couldn't have a White Christmas but, when Greta Engberg dropped in, she suggested that we were having the unique experience of celebrating a Yellow Christmas. At the time, I wasn't especially amused. She also said that if they could find a bright yellow rose to match my skin and put it in my hands, it would make a colorful Kodachrome picture. At that point, I felt quite close to being a colorful corpse. I had lost over thirty pounds and felt miserable.

When I was feeling well enough to be up, I was called to the hospital to see a woman with severe abdominal pain who clearly needed emergency surgery. No other doctor was on hand since Dr. Lofstrom and his family were on vacation. I was in the midst of the operation, removing a twisted ovarian cyst, when a wave of nausea swept over me. My knees buckled and I feared that I might faint. I rushed out just in time and tossed up my breakfast. After a few minutes I returned, re-scrubbed my hands, put on a new sterile gown and gloves, and somehow finished the surgery. I'm pleased to report that my patient recovered from surgery and did not get hepatitis. Obviously, my own battle against the virus hadn't been completely won. I went home and crawled back into bed. Dr. Stan Moris came from the leprosarium to check things out. He ordered me to stay on my back indefinitely.

A few days later, the Lofstroms returned from vacation with Dort at the wheel of the Volkswagen van and Dr. Denny slumped in the passenger seat ill with hepatitis. She was near term with her sixth pregnancy. They had anticipated that I would deliver the baby but when she went into labor a week later, Dennis was in better shape than I was. So—he was called upon to deliver his child, a lovely baby girl to be named Shawn Marie.

When Dort became very ill with hepatitis, we were quite concerned about her for several days until she began recovering. Throughout her illness, she breast-fed little Shawn, who remained well and thrived, never showing any signs of hepatitis.

Our gamma globulin shots didn't seem to have any protective value because new cases of hepatitis occurred in many of those who had received them. Dan was one of these but did not become seriously ill. Then Martha developed a faint yellow tinge in the whites of her eyes and slight darkening of the urine. She didn't even lose her appetite. Adeline was well but exhausted from being a full-time nurse for the rest of us, not to mention teaching Dan and Mark Renner who came to our house from the boarding school when he developed hepatitis.

Since she was still being exposed, Adeline was given another gamma globulin injection. In less than a week she, too, turned yellow and had to go to bed for ten days. That meant that all six of our family had succumbed to the nasty bug. We suspected that the South African gamma globulin didn't contain antibodies against our particular species of hepatitis virus.

The only healthy physician, Dr. Stan Moris, insisted that he wouldn't get hepatitis because he had had it many years before as an intern in Minnesota. Later, he too turned yellow so all four of the mission doctors were down at the same time.

Our African medical assistants and our nurses did a fine job of running the hospital in our absence. Altogether over forty of us became victims of the epidemic. All of us eventually recovered. Dort Lofstrom and I were the most seriously ill. For a few days the doctors had concerns that we might not make it. I lost another ten pounds and never regained my strength during our last year in Africa. It took another year after we returned to America for my liver function tests to return to normal.

16. "BUT DOCTOR! I NEED THE MEDICINE OF THE NEEDLE!"

One morning at Kiomboi Hospital a spry, white-haired, gentleman named Msengi was ushered into my office. He was coughing and had a slight fever but didn't appear to be very sick. I found that he had an upper respiratory infection but no evidence of pneumonia or other significant complications. We gave him some cough medicine and a few aspirins to ease his symptoms. He wasn't at all satisfied with the treatment, declaring, "Lakini Daktari! Ninahitaji *dawa ya sindano!*" (But Doctor! I need the medicine of the needle). His reaction reminded me of another old patient of mine back in Minnesota who came in to see me in the clinic and proclaimed, "Hey Doc, I just got a cold and decided to come in for a shot of penicillin!" Neither one of these patients, 8,000 miles apart, got their requested injections, but it is easy to understand the logic of their demands. Perhaps the Tanganyikan more than the Minnesotan had reason to believe in the supernatural power of the needle.

Even before the days of penicillin, Msengi had witnessed the white medicine man's sorcery brought to Africa in the form of the hypodermic syringe. When he was a young man in the 1930s, many people were afflicted by a horribly disfiguring and debilitating disease known as yaws. Some of the victims were from his own family. The illness is caused by corkscrew-shaped bacteria in the same family as syphilis. It is spread by skin contact in hot humid tropical environments.

Those infected first develop ugly raspberry-textured running sores, and then painful deformed bones and joints which may plague them for the rest of their lives. Soon after the turn of the century, German doctors discovered that injection of certain drugs containing bismuth and arsenic kill the germs causing yaws. The British Colonial Medical services mounted a campaign to eradicate the disease in Tanganyika. In cooperation with medical missionaries, they treated the patients in Msengi's village. After a few injections of arsphenamine, the ulcers melted away and the victims could begin life anew. One happy girl declared that she felt like a butterfly which had come out of an ugly cocoon. Another said that it was like taking off an evil mask. They were astounded and awed by such seemingly supernatural healing.

The success in yaws eradication greatly enhanced the image of Western medicine in the eyes of the Africans. It was discovered that the same arsenical compounds quickly cured another scary disease, tick-borne relapsing fever. Injectable quinine saved babies dying from malaria. The Africans were excited when they saw that smallpox vaccination effectively halted the spread of that terrible malady. All of this happened before the days of sulfa and penicillin. There were therefore several ways in which the *dawa ya sindano* (medicine of the needle) could work its magic. But none was more dramatic in the eyes of the Tanganyikans than the wiping out of yaws. Msengi had witnessed these miracles and concluded that if our injections could melt away such a horrible disease, they could surely do away with his cough and fever.

These developments paved the way for acceptance of Western medicine but they didn't make the populace lose faith in their medicine men. Frequently they sought the wagangas' advice first and came to us only if things weren't going well. We could often tell that we were second choice healers by observing scarification marks on our patients' bodies. Scarification was the medicine man's technique which was most comparable to our medicine of the needle. This treatment consisted of making tiny cuts with a sharp knife over the painful site. If a person had had a headache, there would be fresh cuts or scars on the temples in front of the ears. Many of our adult patients had scarification marks over the spleen because they had experienced pain and swelling there with an attack of malaria. Hepatitis and other liver ailments were treated with scarification over that organ.

The childhood segment of the Iramba population did not appreciate our hypodermic needles. Giving injections, drawing blood, or doing spinal taps on innocent little ones has always been my least favorite facet of pediatrics. (Of course, I usually had the nurses do most of my dirty work while I closed my eyes and held my hands over my ears!) The African mothers were very good about restraining their little ones and seeing that they received the recommended needling. I suspect they, like some American mothers, also used the threat of shots to coerce improved behavior in their offspring.

We doctors weren't above using that weapon ourselves. In Africa I never resorted to a trick I once used on an American child. One day in the waiting room of my private office in Colorado a five-year-old patient was conducting a one-boy riot. He was screaming, yelling, and tearing the place apart and his mother was unable to control him. On impulse, I formulated a sneaky strategic battle plan. I attached a monstrous five-inch spinal needle to a huge syringe about an inch in diameter and six inches long. Then I filled it with nasty looking green antiseptic solution and placed it on an instrument tray. Like a waiter in a restaurant serving up the main dish, I carried the tray from the emergency room through the waiting area past my rampaging patient and back into my office. (He and his mother were the only occupants of the reception room at the time). I made sure that our little rebel saw my awesome weapon but didn't say a word. When he spotted it, his jaw dropped and he immediately walked quietly over to sit in his mother's lap. She smiled and gave me the thumbs up sign. Later when she led him meekly into my examining room, he was a little pale. Fortunately, I was able to reassure him that he wasn't going to get any shot that day and we became good buddies.

Another magical property of our needles was their ability to relieve and prevent pain. When I removed a small tumor from the leg of my medicine man friend, Ntindilo, I used Novocain injection. He was astounded and just couldn't get over the fact that there was no hurting.

No dentists practiced in Irambaland so I was sometimes called upon to pull badly decayed teeth. I had learned the rudiments of dental anesthesia using Novocain. Several of my patients were relieved to discover that having a tooth pulled didn't have to be the agonizing ordeal with which they were only too familiar. We used spinal anesthesia frequently because it was safer than deep inhalation anesthesia in our setting. This was frightening to our African patients, and we had to keep reassuring them that they would soon regain sensation and the use of their legs. On some occasions we also used intravenous barbiturates to induce sleep before surgery. This too was amazing to those who had never experienced or witnessed anything like it. All of these modes of preventing pain added to the mystical aura surrounding our medicine of the needle.

One final episode portrays both the gratification and the frustration of my own opportunities to introduce the *dawa ya sindano* in places where it had never been experienced. I was on a hunting expedition with two African friends about twenty miles out on the plains. We drove near the small temporary village of a nomadic cattle-herding tribe. A young man bearing a wicked-looking spear came out of one of the huts and ran towards our jeep. I was a little apprehensive until we saw that he was desperately trying to wave us down. In Swahili he indicated that the headman of their group was very sick.

I grabbed the small medical emergency bag which I always carried in the Jeep. I followed him to one of the huts and he motioned me to enter. I had to stoop low to get through the door which was no more than four feet in height. In the dim half-light I saw a middle-aged man who was struggling to get his breath and wheezing loudly. He had been fine until an hour earlier when he had had a coughing attack which gradually led to his present distress. With my stethoscope I could hear the typical wheezing of a severe asthma attack. He had previously experienced similar episodes. The chief had never been to a Western medical facility in his life. Tribal medicine men had given him herbal preparations which gave some relief. In my kit I had a vial of adrenalin and sterile syringes. I injected the appropriate dose into his arm, and then we waited. Within five minutes his wheezing almost disappeared. I'll never forget his smile of surprise and relief as he looked first at me and then the syringe which I was still holding.

The response was gratifying but I was frustrated in having to tell him that the magic medicine would only last about two hours. If he came to our hospital, we could give him some pills which would afford longer relief, but I wasn't certain that they would be much better than the leaves which his tribal medicine man could furnish him. After all, our asthma medications were passed down to us by our ancestral medicine men and we hadn't improved on them very much. In the 1950s we simply didn't have surefire effective preparations to manage asthma. The medicine of the needle was powerful but it couldn't deal effectively with all health problems.

17. "MY TOOTH HURTS!"

The closest practicing dentist to Irambaland was two hundred miles away in Arusha. Most of our African patients had no concept as to what a dentist was or did. They assumed that since we mission doctors dealt with the problems of the entire body we should be able to care for their mouths and teeth. When they had painful dental problems, they didn't hesitate to come to our hospitals or clinics.

We did not have a high incidence of dental decay in our population, probably because refined sugar wasn't readily available. Sugar cane wasn't cultivated in Central Tanganyika as it was in other regions. In communities where it was grown, children chewed on it continuously, developing terrible dental decay. The cattle-herding tribes including the Masai and the Barabaig had conspicuously beautiful teeth. Their diet was primarily made up of the meat, milk and blood from their cattle, sheep and goats.

Dr. Martin Aliker, a Ugandan graduate of Northwestern University Dental School, spoke to us about childhood dental health at the UNICEF conference in Kampala. His studies indicated that African children in Uganda had less dental decay than European children. He felt that the amount and frequency of exposure to refined sugar was the difference.

Many African ethnic groups have a tradition of making a toothbrush by chewing on the small branch of a certain tree. They brush regularly and seem to get rid of a lot of the debris around their teeth. We saw this practice often in Kiomboi and Iambi. Some African groups practiced rinsing their mouths with water after meals which would be the next best thing to brushing the teeth.

Fluoride content of the ground water made a significant difference in dental health. The tribal areas of the Kikuyu in

Kenya and the Wachagga in Tanganyika had high water fluoride content which caused an orange staining of the teeth. We saw this discoloration occasionally in Irambaland but had no information about the fluoride in our water. We probably had a protective amount since little tooth decay occurred in our Iramba-Turu population.

The most common dental problem in Iramba adults was periodontal or gum disease. In many instances the gums receded from the roots until eventually teeth loosened and fell out.

Some of our people still ground their corn or millet on grinding stones. The flour thus produced contained tiny rock particles which over long periods wore the teeth down severely. It was easy to recognize because their teeth were abraded right down into the root canals with painful complications.

We mission doctors and nurses avoided promoting our dental capabilities. We were, however, called upon to do what we could to relieve pain. Each of our hospitals had a dental kit for emergencies. Oil of cloves applied with a cotton ball directly into an open cavity gave relief of much of the pain. I also repaired several gaping holes with temporary fillings which often stayed in place for several months.

Frequently we were called upon to pull decayed teeth. Our supply cabinets contained basic instruments for dental extraction. I had learned to inject Novocain into the lower jaw at the point where the nerve comes out of the bone. Such a nerve block gives almost complete relief from pain and makes pulling a tooth much easier for both the puller and the pullee. I became fairly adept at this technique, making a number of successful extractions.

I was becoming a little complacent at my tooth-pulling prowess when I was brought back down to earth by a humiliating experience. A small shopping area was located near

Kiomboi Hospital. One of the dukas (stores) was owned by an East Indian named Manjhi Danjhi. He was prosperous enough to afford dental care. One day he brought his wife into my office with a terrible toothache. Her right lower jaw was swollen and seemed to be developing an abscess. She said that her tooth had been aching for weeks. I scolded her husband, telling him to put her on a bus to Arusha to be treated properly by a dentist. He promised he would, but couldn't I give her something for temporary relief. I looked into her mouth and found a huge cavity in one of the lower molars. I applied oil of cloves into the gaping hole and the poor woman experienced some relief from the awful pain. We also gave her a large injection of long-acting penicillin to control the infection. Mr. Danjhi promised to take her to Arusha where he knew one of the dentists who was a fellow East Indian.

A week later the couple returned because Mrs. Danjhi was in more distress than ever. Manjhi looked a little sheepish as he admitted that he hadn't followed my instructions to get her to Arusha. We couldn't tell whether or not he was too stingy to spend the money or if she was resistant to going that far away from home. She had improved somewhat after the penicillin, but then became worse again. Now wouldn't I just pull that bad tooth and get it over with. I was tempted to send them on their way but felt terribly sorry for her. I decided to get rid of that monstrous molar, much to my later dismay.

We took Mrs. Danjhi into the treatment room and I was able to do a Novocain nerve block on her right lower jaw. When I grasped the badly decayed molar with the forceps, there was an awful crunching sound. I had broken off both the crown of the bad tooth and the good molar next to it! Now I would have to dig out the roots of both teeth. I dug and scraped and pulled unsuccessfully for about an hour. By that time the local anesthesia was wearing off, so I had our nurse-anesthetist give her ether. It took almost another hour to pry out the roots. When she awoke, she found herself missing not only the bad tooth but the good one next to it. Her husband may have been unhappy, but he didn't dare say anything because he knew that I was upset with him.

When we returned to the States, I was happy that I no longer had to worry about pulling or filling teeth.

18. "WHEN ARE YOU GOING TO GIVE ME THE REAL TREATMENT?"

When I was a barefoot boy in the Ozarks, my mother frequently expressed fear of her children stepping on a thorn or nail and getting lockjaw. In her childhood she had experienced the death of a school friend who had punctured her foot on a wooden splinter.

In medical school I saw only one case of tetanus. A small child was admitted to St. Louis Children's Hospital with that dreaded diagnosis and given all of the available treatment. We medical students watched in horror and anguished with the parents as this child died a horrible death over the next two weeks. Our brilliant professors were unable to alter the downhill course.

Tetanus was well known in Tanganyika. I didn't have to wait long for my first encounter. A young man named Mkumbo was brought to the hospital from his home several miles away.

Four male relatives carefully set down the wooden bed upon which they were carrying him. The impact of his cot touching the floor with a slight jarring sound triggered a terrible spasm of his entire body. Mkumbo's neck and back were arched sharply backwards, with arms partially extended and his fingers drawn up like claws. An inhuman groan was followed by a desperate effort to breathe. His facial muscles were locked in a grotesque smile which doctors have described for centuries with the Latin words, risus sardonicus. All the muscles of his body were frozen in a rock-hard involuntary contraction. For at least a minute he was unable to breathe and his lips assumed an ominous blue color. Finally, there was a gradual relaxation and resumption of shallow noisy respiration. We had difficulty in opening his mouth to clear out his respiratory secretions. It was easy to see why the term lockjaw had been applied to such an ailment. We carefully carried him into the hospital and laid him on a bed.

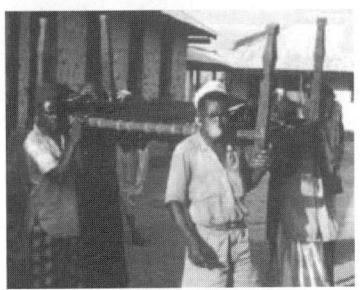

African ambulance

As I examined him further, I noted several strange pea-sized nodules on his feet. I recognized them as Chigoe flea burrows, or funzas as they were called in Swahili. They resembled blisters with tiny central holes. Through a magnifying glass, I could see clusters of almost microscopic shiny white eggs coming out of the pinhead-sized openings. Each funza is formed by a pregnant female flea burrowing between the layers of skin and setting up housekeeping and propagation.

The openings also provide ideal invasion channels for bacteria. Tetanus-producing germs can only grow in enclosed environments with limited oxygen where they produce the toxin which is one of the most powerful poisons known to man. In our patient, a badly inflamed funza was almost certainly the point of origin of his tetanus.

Our immediate problem was to keep our patient alive. He was desperately ill with violent spasms every few minutes. In between attacks, his respiration was shallow and labored. He hadn't been able to eat for several days and his liquid intake was poor, resulting in dehydration. We gave him a large dose of tetanus antitoxin. Unfortunately, this doesn't counteract the poison already fixed to the nerve-muscle endings but neutralizes the toxin still floating in the bloodstream. Tranquilizing, muscle-relaxing medications were given to reduce the intensity of the recurring spasms. Fluids and nourishment were given through a tube in one nostril and down into the stomach. I carefully cleaned out the Chigoe flea burrows on his feet and began treatment with antibiotics. We assigned one of our nurses to watch him constantly, to suck out the secretions in his throat and be aware of any ominous developments. On that first day, I didn't expect him to survive.

For the next three days there was no improvement. If anything, he seemed worse. Although he was conscious and aware of what was happening, the spasm of his throat muscles prevented him from talking. I still didn't believe that he was going to make it. About the fifth day one of our medical assistants said, "I think Mkumbo is a little better this morning." The hospital chart did indicate that his spasms were less frequent. He tried to tell us something but still couldn't articulate well enough for us to understand. From that day on, he showed daily improvement.

About the tenth day as I was examining him, Mkumbo grasped my arm and said what could be translated as, "When are you going to give me the real treatment, Doctor?"

I was totally flabbergasted. Here he was, clearly on the road to recovery, but we had obviously not fulfilled his expectations. I tried to explain that the injections, medications, and other treatments we had done were all that was necessary for him to become completely well again.

"But," he replied, "You haven't gotten rid of the evil spirit!"

I tried to explain that our medicines would chase away the bad spirits. He looked at me tolerantly, as if this poor mzungu Daktari simply couldn't fathom the real facts of life. I then asked him what the 'real treatment' should be. Mkumbo explained that we had to kill a white goat and go through an elaborate ritual to exorcise the evil spirit. I stuck to my original contention that further measures were unnecessary. For the next three days he kept after me, but I stubbornly refused to add the white goat to our treatment program. Perhaps an older, wiser doctor would have seen a way through this impasse. I just couldn't see why my patient needed the sacrifice of a white goat when he had a bright young doctor wearing a white coat!

By this time he was able to sit up in bed and could stand with difficulty. He was still having occasional spasms which would temporarily immobilize him. He certainly wasn't ready to go home, but in the middle of the night he disappeared. We didn't know where he lived and never saw him again.

I suspect that Mkumbo went straight to the local medicine man and underwent the complete white goat ritual. I asked several of our African staff why he wasn't satisfied with the obvious physical recovery which followed our treatment. The most plausible explanation came from one of our medical assistants. He indicated that the Iramba people recognize the symptoms of tetanus and are convinced that it is caused by bewitchment. Even if the disease is not severe, they are certain that it will be fatal if the hex is not lifted. Usually they went to the medicine man first, and then came to our hospital if things weren't going well. Mkumbo apparently came to the hospital first. Although he recognized that he was improving, our methods didn't satisfy the criteria dictated by strong indigenous cultural persuasions.

One of our Christian Iramba friends told me that if he had tetanus he didn't think that he would have Mkumbo's problem because he believed that his faith would overcome the evil spirit. Then he wryly shook his head and admitted that if things weren't going well in the hospital he would be tempted to call in the mganga, too. Western doctors with many years' experience in Africa acknowledge that indigenous medicine men have many astounding success stories in treating patients desperately ill with tetanus. Perhaps if we paid more attention to their methods and medications we would learn something.

Over the next four years I participated in the treatment of twenty-five more patients who clearly had tetanus. Of these, only one died, a newborn with an ugly umbilical cord infection. She was brought in with terrible spasms and far advanced pneumonia. She died before we could initiate treatment. Our mortality rate was much lower than that reported at the time in America. This was definitely not a tribute to our medical skills because we were functioning under very primitive conditions. One theory was that our patients had partially immunized themselves by going barefoot for their first years in an environment around cattle heavily populated by tetanus-producing germs. Tiny cracks in the skin of the feet could permit non-lethal exposure with production of some antibodies to the tetanus toxin. This hypothesis has not been proven. Most of our twenty-six lockjaw patients had infected wounds which were the likely points of entry of the tetanus-causing bacteria. Nine of them had Chigoe flea burrows on their feet.

Our American mission family was well aware of the hazards of going barefoot or wearing sandals in funza territory. Several missionaries had to dig out the nasty little creatures from their feet. Fortunately we didn't have to send our children barefoot through the corral to give them a little immunity from lockjaw. DPT shots in early childhood and a tetanus booster every ten years provide almost foolproof protection against this dreadful disease.

19. LEPROSY

Some of my most gratifying experiences in Africa occurred while working with our leprosy patients. Most of them were cheerful, uncomplaining, and remarkably self-sufficient. In spite of grotesque deformities and staggering disabilities, they tended to smile frequently and make the best of difficult situations.

The word leprosy, now known as Hansen's disease, has generated horror and repugnance in the minds of men for thousands of years. It is caused by slow-growing bacteria of the same family as tuberculosis. Only about 5 percent of individuals intimately exposed ever develop the disease. An average incubation is three to five years, but in rare instances leprosy becomes apparent as long as thirty years after known exposure. The bacilli grow primarily in the skin, superficial nerves, and mucous membranes of the nose and upper respiratory tracts.

The most common skin manifestations are de-pigmented patches with a loss of sensation. Often the first awareness comes with anesthesia of the hands or feet whereupon the victim burns, or otherwise damages, fingers or toes because he feels no pain. Repeated injuries of the sensation-less extremities ultimately result in the serious deformities of the hands and feet. The small muscles of the hands become paralyzed and wither away. Fingers and toes don't just drop off. The bones are gradually dissolved with shortening of the digits. It is not unusual to see a patient with a row of fingernails just beyond the knuckles which makes the hands resemble animal paws.

The different types of leprosy are determined by the victim's immune response to the bacteria. About 80 percent of our African patients had tuberculoid leprosy. In this type, bodies mount an active defense against the germs invading their skin and nerve tissue. The immune system succeeds in killing most of the germs but the inflammation required to do so also destroys the nerve fibers. The bacteria are eliminated but the damage is beyond repair.

Lepromatous leprosy, with the horrible lumpy facial deformities, is most often pictured in lay publications. Only about 10 percent of our Iramba patients had this type in which the body seems to be defenseless; the bacilli multiply unchecked in the skin, nerves, and mucous membranes. When observed under the microscope, skin smears are teeming with leprosy bacilli.

The lines between tuberculoid and lepromatous leprosy weren't always clear-cut. In such cases the term indeterminate was applied.

The social stigma of leprosy in Africa was similar to that of most cultures throughout human history. Once the disease was recognized in a person, he became an outcast. Those infected were expected to go away and live with others with leprosy. The disease was legitimate grounds for divorce, but spouses often chose to remain with their afflicted husbands or wives.

When missionaries first arrived, they found leprosy settlements scattered through the countryside. Often these were situated in the least desirable locations with pitiful living conditions and a lack of social cohesiveness. When the British assumed leadership of the country, they tried to help, but other priorities minimized their accomplishments. Medical missionaries and international organizations such as the British Red Cross and American Leprosy Mission assumed much of the responsibility for the care of this long-suffering population.

Surveys had indicated that the incidence of leprosy in the Iramba-Turu area was 1.5 to 2 percent. This added up to a total of about five thousand Hansen's disease patients for which we were responsible. In 1957 we were taking care of approximately five hundred of them. Much more work needed to be done.

Dr. Stanley Moris, a veteran of many years of service in both China and Africa, was assigned to work full-time in the leprosy program. For years he had made careful studies of the disease and visited treatment programs in America, the Orient, and India.

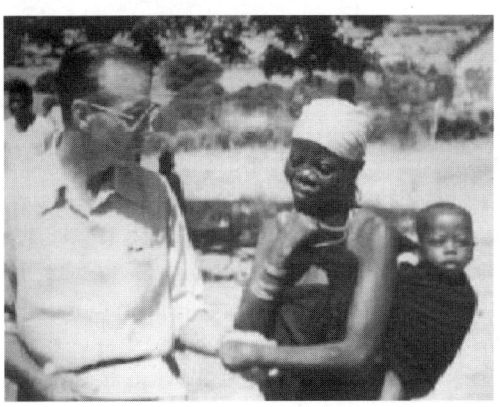

Dr. Stan Moris with patient

With the financial assistance and consultation of the American Leprosy Mission and government medical authorities, Dr. Stan had formulated well-defined plans for an up-to-date hospital, rehabilitation center and residential community. A large unoccupied tract was chosen five miles east of our

Iambi Hospital. I had brought home impala and wildebeest for our refrigerator from this prime hunting area.

Construction had begun under the supervision of a British contractor, Stan Alderson. Some of the patients from the Mkalama leprosy colony had settled in to make up his work crew. Dr. Moris was due to go home on furlough soon after my arrival, so it would be up to me to deal with the medical problems of the leprosy patients. I was apprehensive but felt better in knowing that two experienced American nurses, Helen Erickson and Greta Ekstrand, were on hand. Under Stan's tutelage, I took a crash course in diagnosis, laboratory studies, treatment, and the daily management of common leprosy problems.

We had an adequate supply of the sulfone drugs which had revolutionized treatment over the previous decade. When given twice weekly this medication effectively eliminated the leprosy bacillus from those infected. Unfortunately, it occasionally precipitated painful reactions with fever, pain, and bizarre rashes which needed to be watched closely.

Iambi Leprosarium was being developed on land which had not been previously occupied because there was no year-round water supply. Arrangements were made for a young British water resources engineer, John Holloway, to plan and construct an earthen dam which would produce a permanent lake of several acres. This project took several months to complete. John often stayed at our house when he was at Iambi and became a great favorite of our children. The work was finished just before the monsoon season. When the rains came and the reservoir started to fill, we were all delighted.

One night four-year-old Dan had just said his prayers at bedtime and was making some thoughtful commentaries on things as he saw them. He declared, "God makes the mountains and John Holloway makes the lakes!"

Incidentally, John was later to become one of the main engineers on the huge project to prevent the Thames River tides from flooding London. A complex system of dams, dikes, channels and water gates has been constructed to prevent excessively high waters from North Sea storms and tides from rushing up the river as far as London. John was honored in being selected to escort Queen Elizabeth through the project on Dedication Day.

Now that we had a reliable water source, more families moved in from the outlying leprosy villages to construct their homes and plant their crops. At this point, our agricultural missionary, Roland Renner, arrived on the scene with his family. He made an immediate contribution in helping the patients establish new homes and grow their own foods. The tractor which he brought made gardens possible for those who were too disabled to till the virgin soil with their hoes. We were amazed at how much the patients with claw hands and stump feet could do for themselves, but they were thrilled to have the hard clay turned over with a plow. Roly also introduced tomatoes, beans, carrots, eggplant and other good vegetables which significantly improved nutrition. He was instrumental in assisting them in establishing a communally owned herd of cattle.

Roly was also called upon to destroy an opportunistic twenty-foot python which had discovered that our reservoir was a great place to ambush small animals and perhaps even children. A few days later a dozen baby pythons appeared in the same corner of the reservoir. They had apparently been produced by the big mama before her demise. These were also destroyed because little snakes later become big ones. In many different ways Roly, his wife Marge, and their four lively sons helped make Iambi Leprosarium a happy new home for the patients and their families.

Friends and family in America were shocked to learn that our missionary children were often in close contact with leprosy patients. On some occasions, our children had to sit next to a patient we were transporting in a jeep. The four young Renner boys were in contact with leprosy patients every day. We were diligent in keeping the children away from infectious patients, and they were taught early on that they must wash their hands carefully.

A question often asked of us who worked with leprosy patients has been, "Weren't you afraid of getting the disease yourselves?" The example of Father Damien, the Belgian priest, was often cited. In 1885 he developed leprosy after he dedicated his life to those suffering from the disease at the infamous Molokai colony in Hawaii. Our answer to such queries was, "In all the years our medical workers, pastors, and teachers of all races have been in close contact with infectious cases in Tanzania, not one of us has developed Hansen's disease." Of course we were careful, especially when dealing with those with untreated lepromatous disease.

Intimate skin contact seemed to be the predominate mode of infection in our patients. Often the first patch of the disease in African children appeared on the foreheads of those whose mothers had communicable leprosy. These little ones rode on their mothers' backs and rubbed their foreheads back and forth against her germ-laden skin. Several years later a telltale white patch suggested the mode of infection.

Other factors besides skin contact determined whether or not a person would develop leprosy. Far less leprosy developed in populations with a good high-protein diet. Dr. Moris reported that he had never seen a case of leprosy among our Barabaig patients. This cattle-herding nomadic tribe lived off the meat, milk, and blood of their livestock, much like the

Masai. We don't know why they seemed immune to leprosy. It is uncertain whether the diet or genetic factors gave them some resistance.

In 1958 our family took a two-week vacation in the beautiful green Southern Highlands of Tanganyika. This 1000-mile safari over primitive roads in a jeep truck would also make it possible for me to visit the well-established Makete Leprosarium near Mbeya. Makete was located in a fertile valley. The population density was higher than in Irambaland because of the rich volcanic soil and generous rainfall. The incidence of leprosy was also high. Hopefully, I would be able to observe and learn practical measures which would be of use to us at Iambi. At the same time we could be enjoying one of the most picturesque regions of East Africa.

The Makete leprosy program had been generously funded by the British Red Cross and had an international staff. As we were nearing the leprosarium we had to stop twice to ask directions from Africans walking along the road. Each time they greeted us in the traditional friendly Swahili manner, except that they didn't say, "Jambo!" The pronunciation was distinctly, "Yambo, Bwana!" When we finally arrived at our destination, we were met by a cheerful blonde woman who welcomed us with a hearty, "Yambo! Yambo!" The Africans who had directed us earlier had probably sized us up as Scandihoovians and used what they thought was the appropriate pronunciation in their salutations. We soon discovered that our hostess, Rigmor Hansen, was straight out of Denmark. She helped us settle into the rustic but comfortable guest house.

We spent two full but relaxing days at Makete. The community was made up of over 1,000 leprosy patients and their families. Most were not infectious but still had deformities which were being treated with surgery, plus physical and occupational therapy. Virtually all of them were living in thatched African style homes which they themselves had built. All but the most crippled raised their own food: vegetables, chickens and small livestock,. In all outward appearances, Makete was a happy and well functioning community.

The British doctor who was in charge took me on rounds through the hospital wards which included an active obstetrics unit. I was intrigued to observe the procedure for babies delivered from mothers with infectious leprosy. The little ones were kept in a separate nursery for the first two years of life and brought to their mamas when it was time to nurse. Each of the babies was wrapped in a large cotton muslin bag to limit the skin contact which might infect the baby.

If the mother was still infectious as determined by skin smears, the child would be given prophylactic sulfone drugs by mouth for two more years. Research studies suggested that these rather heroic efforts were reducing the number of new cases of leprosy among the babies in the bags. I felt sorry for the mothers as I watched them trying to cuddle their little sacks of humanity.

Our Danish nurse Rigmor took me on a tour of the outlying village clinics where many non-infectious patients were being treated without having to leave their home environment. It was already anticipated that with the success of control programs, so-called leprosy colonies would be unnecessary in a few years. The use of more soap and water and improved nutrition also was having an impact on limiting the spread of leprosy.

The Makete community had a large primary school made up mostly of children of patients. A few of the students had early signs of the disease of the non-communicable type and many of them were on prophylactic sulfone drugs because of their parents' disease. On the last day of our visit, we were honored with an exciting parade by about sixty of the students lined up in four columns. Leading the way was a proud little baton-bearing drum major about ten years of age with early signs of leprosy. He sported a red fez cap and a bright pink sash draped across his uniform of khaki shirt and shorts. Just behind him, four boys marched along beating a snappy cadence on their homemade African drums. Their performance was one of the happiest and most emotionally moving parades I had ever witnessed. These young students symbolized the anticipation of a brighter future for a population which a few years earlier had lived without hope in grim isolation and disgrace.

Progress accelerated at Iambi when Dr. Moris came back from his furlough. He was assisted by an excellent staff of Africans and missionaries. One valuable addition was Lore Heidel, a refugee from East Germany who was trained in both physical and occupational therapy. The outstanding nursing staff included my sister Veda who had an extensive experience during her first four years at the Tintigulu leprosy village on the Wembere Plains. Great sadness enveloped our mission family and African coworkers when one of the leprosarium nurses, Lavinia Holcomb, was killed by a propane stove explosion. Another nurse, Lois Bernhardson, who was trained in laboratory procedures, became a vital member of the team. Agriculturist Rolly Renner and his family contributed in many ways to the success of the program. In every aspect of the work, Dr. Stan's wife Edith was an invaluable member of the team.

All of the staff, both African and American, developed a healthy camaraderie and a deep caring commitment to their patients. Working together, they literally transformed the lives of hundreds of Hansen's disease victims and their families at Iambi Leprosarium. They also set up a system of outpatient clinics to find new cases and to enable many victims to remain in their home villages.

After my first year at Iambi, I was transferred to Kiomboi Hospital, but I eagerly followed developments at the leprosarium and visited as often as possible. Now, many years later, when I look back at my leprosy experience, one of the first people who come to mind is Musa. He developed severe leprosy in his teen years and was ostracized by his clan. Until he came to Iambi, he lived in a dismal village with fellow victims. He was already totally blind when I first met him. The invading bacilli had destroyed the cartilage of his face and larynx, collapsing his nose and giving his voice a harsh nasal quality. His hands and feet were so terribly deformed that he could barely hobble around, but he never complained. Whenever I greeted him and asked him how he was, he invariably responded with a big smile and a cheerful, "I'm just fine, Daktari!"

Musa and Veda were good buddies and had many friendly visits. One day she was in a hurry to get to the hospital for an emergency. She walked past Musa without greeting him as he sat in the sunshine outside his home on the path to the hospital. She assumed that being blind he wouldn't be aware of her presence. But just after she passed, he called in an aggrieved voice, "Aren't you even going to say hello to me, Bibi Veda?" Somewhat startled by his apparent extrasensory perception, she asked him, "Musa! How did you know that I was here?" With a grin and a twinkle in his blind eyes he replied, "I smelled your soap!"

Thirty years after I had first worked at Iambi, we returned for a visit. Iambi Leprosarium was no more, having been developed into a 300-bed general hospital. Practically all of the leprosy patients had either been cured or returned to their home communities for outpatient treatment. The open savanna where I had hunted wild game was now thickly populated with people. We arrived at Iambi late at night in a heavy monsoon rain and were welcomed warmly by Dr. David Dyauli. He had been one of our finest Medical Assistants in 1957, had gone on to medical school in Dar es Salaam, and was now the doctor in charge of the hospital. He welcomed us into his home which had once been the abode of Dr. and Mrs. Moris. In the absence of his wife, Dr. Dyauli indicated that his lovely nineteen-year-old daughter would be our hostess. He smiled as he told us that her name was Adeline and that she had been named after Bibi Hult. Over the years we had corresponded several times but David had never mentioned that my Adeline had a namesake in Africa. That was a pleasant surprise and the two Adelines developed a special rapport during our two day visit.

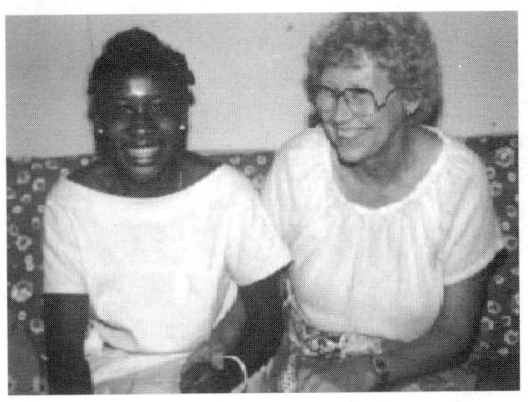

Adeline Daudi and Adeline Hult

The following day after the morning devotional service in the chapel we were happily greeted by eight African staff members with whom I had worked. They proudly gave us a complete tour of the hospital. We did not see any leprosy patients until we reached the last ward which contained three elderly gentlemen. I immediately recognized one of them as our "I-know-you-by-the-smell-of-your-soap!" friend Musa. He didn't identify me by my odor, but as soon as he heard my voice, he flashed a beaming smile of recognition. Other than having white hair and being a little heavier, he was the same old Musa. When I asked him how he was, he responded with his trademark smile and a cheery, "Mzuri sana!" which translates into, "Just great!" He was glad to see me but was much more interested in catching up on the news of his friend, Veda. He was happy to hear that she was in good health, but wondered plaintively why she hadn't come back to Iambi. I told him that she had married a widowed pastor with four children and was very busy. He indicated that he still missed her.

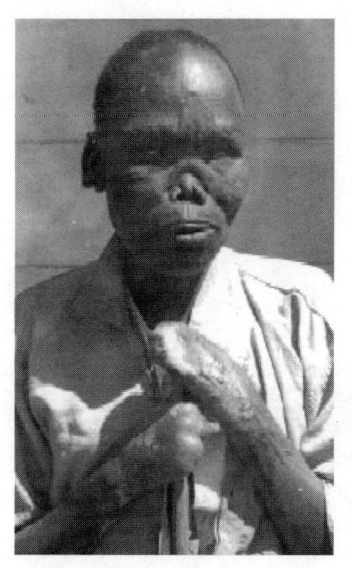

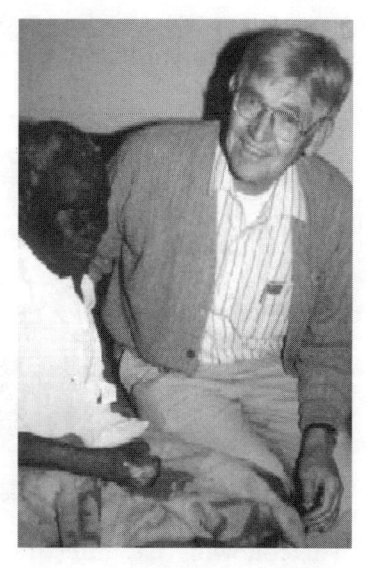

Musa - 1957 *Musa and Daktari Yohana, 1987*

After saying goodbye to Musa, our last stop was at the outpatient clinic. We found two technicians fitting a custom-built protective shoe on an elderly woman with tuberculoid leprosy. She beamed as she stood up and walked comfortably around the room with her stylish new black leather foot-ware. We also watched a young man getting a form of physiotherapy which consisted of dipping his hand in warm melted paraffin and doing exercises to increase mobility.

The staff hoped that they would be able to get a hand surgeon to come to Iambi to work on some of their patients with claw hands. Dr. Herbert Plock from Germany had performed such restorative surgery on many patients at Iambi from 1966 to 1980. He had learned these techniques in India from missionary surgeon, Dr. Paul Brand. Tendons were transplanted from healthy deep muscles of the forearm to replace those paralyzed in the hands and fingers by leprosy. After surgery some of these patients with completely immobilized hands were able to perform such skilled tasks as playing the piano and typing.

Leprosy work in Irambaland has been a significant success story. The disease is steadily being confined and wiped out. Education has enlightened the population to the extent that the victims are no longer feared and ostracized. Dr. Moris deserves a large measure of credit, but those whom he taught are continuing his good work. Dr. Hosea Namilikwa, with whom I worked while he was still a Medical Assistant, became the Medical officer in charge of tuberculosis and leprosy work in the vast Central Province of Tanzania. It is predicted that in a few more decades leprosy will be as rare in Africa as in the Western world. For me, it was exciting and gratifying to have been on the scene when the action was really intensifying. I feel privileged to have had a small part in the work and to have been the recipient of the gratitude and friendship of people like Musa.

20. UNWELCOME GUESTS

Parasitic diseases play an important role in the overall health of both children and adults in Africa. We frequently discovered that an individual patient harbored several different kinds of worms or other parasites. These opportunistic creatures have figured out effective ways in which to sneak into our bodies and make a living at our expense. Some are quite benign but others become true killers. Fortunately, we have the ability to get rid of most of these little animals, or better, to prevent them from getting into our bodies in the first place.

It would take a thick volume to discuss all of them, but the following stories of patients with parasites illustrate three of the problems we faced.

Selemani, a five-year-old Iramba boy, was brought into the clinic because he was pale, listless, weak, and short of breath. He was pot-bellied, had puffy eyes, and his hemoglobin was less than half of what it should have been. He was seriously ill, with borderline heart failure. A microscopic stool examination revealed large numbers of hookworm eggs and his blood smear showed malaria. We put him in the hospital and first dealt with his malaria. Then we treated him with tetrachlorethylene, which was the most effective medicine available to eradicate hookworm. With supplemental vitamins and iron added to his diet, he slowly made a complete recovery.

This was the first case of severe hookworm disease I had seen in Tanganyika. It is not common in areas with less than forty inches of rainfall. Moist soil is necessary for the survival of hookworm larvae. Selemani's family had a garden near the river where the ground was damp even during the dry season.

He spent a lot of time playing there and obviously had much skin contact with the infected soil.

Hookworm eggs are deposited in the soil with the stools of an infected individual. After hatching, the larvae, which are invisible to the naked eye, enter the body by penetrating the skin and entering tiny blood vessels. They are carried through the right side of the heart to the lung capillaries where they invade the air sacs, crawl into the bronchial tubes, are coughed up and swallowed. As they mature, they attach themselves to the lining of the small intestine. The name hookworm derives from the shark-like teeth around the mouth with which they latch onto the host's intestinal lining. After mating, the males die. The females remain attached and may live for up to fifteen years, each one laying 10,000 to 20,000 eggs per day. This longevity was determined by a parasitologist who allowed himself to be infected with hookworm larvae. With no possibilities of re-infection, he was still finding the eggs in his stools after fifteen years.

Female hookworms are voracious feeders. Although they are only one-third inch long, a light infection of sixty worms can consume an ounce of blood per day. That would add up to a quart every month. Heavy hookworm infections can and do kill. This was first realized in Switzerland in 1880 when a number of miners digging the famous St. Gothard Tunnel died of overwhelming hookworm disease. The earth in which they were working was massively contaminated with larvae from careless stool deposits by infected laborers.

Hookworm is not just a disease of the tropics. At one time in our own Southern states the Public Health Department determined that there were over two million cases. Fortunately, sanitary disposal of human waste has greatly reduced the problem in the United States. Also, the simple practice of wearing shoes keeps the larvae away from the skin, thereby preventing infection even when the soil is contaminated.

In Tanganyika we found at least a few hookworm eggs in one third of all the patients tested, but only a small minority of these had anemia. Apparently, healthy individuals who are continuously exposed develop a degree of immunity which doesn't eliminate all larvae but prevents overwhelming infection.

A young African cattle herder named Msengi came to our clinic one day complaining of painful urination. His urine was tinged red with blood. He had also had intermittent fever for several weeks with poor appetite and loss of strength. An examination revealed that his liver and spleen were enlarged, and there was tenderness over his bladder. A specimen of his urine contained the eggs of Schistosoma hematobium. A few months earlier he had begun taking his livestock to a new water hole. Every day, while the cattle were drinking, he went into the water to bathe and cool off. We asked him if he knew other people with the same symptoms. He replied that several friends who used this water source had similar complaints.

It was clear that Msengi had schistosomiasis, a serious and debilitating chronic disease caused by worm-like parasites which live in the small veins draining the bladder and lower intestinal tract. It is widespread in Africa, especially in countries such as Egypt where irrigation is practiced. Two species of the parasite, S. hematobium and S. mansoni, live in the small veins of the bladder and those of the lower intestinal tract respectively.

The adults are from one-third to two-thirds of an inch in length. The stocky male holds the slender female in a permanent embrace. His grotesque front end includes a mouth on the end of an elephant-like trunk, behind which lies a disc-shaped sucker with which he grips the inside of the vein in which he and his mate live. The adults may live from twenty to thirty years. The microscopic eggs from an infected human host are passed either in urine or feces into water where they hatch into a free-swimming stage which invade certain species of freshwater snails. After multiplying and developing into an infective tadpole-shaped stage called cercaria, they leave the snails in large numbers and return to the water where they await a human victim. They penetrate the skin and are carried through the blood vessels to the liver. After maturing, they migrate against the flow of blood to the small veins of the bladder or lower intestine where they pair off and begin their years of procreation.

Most of the damage in humans is produced by the eggs which are deposited in the tissue of the bladder and intestinal tract and are also carried to the liver, spleen, and lungs where they produce serious debilitating inflammation and scarring. Schistosomiasis is also associated with an increased incidence of cancer of the bladder and liver.

The outlook is good for an individual with schistosomiasis if treated early and further infection is avoided. We treated Msengi with Stibophen, an antimony-containing compound which effectively kills the adult parasites, and we urged him to stay out of the contaminated water hole. In far advanced cases, treatment produces little improvement because the damage is irreversible.

Schistosomiasis is actually a more serious and challenging public health problem than malaria in affected countries. Much research has been done on developing a vaccine. Efforts to eradicate the snail hosts have had limited success and may lead to serious ecological complications. An article in the November 1994 Discover Magazine reported an intriguing investigation being conducted in Kenya. Louisiana crayfish, which were already being grown in Africa as a potential source of dietary protein, have been shown to voraciously feed on snails. It is hoped that their introduction to waters harboring schistosome parasites might reduce the snail population enough to make an impact on the incidence of the disease. Keeping people out of the water isn't feasible when it is their only source for drinking, bathing, washing, and irrigation. Education and improved public health should eventually eliminate this disease, but that is probably decades away.

Over the years several of our missionaries in Tanzania have had to be treated during the early stages of schistosomiasis. Our family carefully avoided wading or bathing in any body of water which might harbor the parasites. Sometimes our children didn't understand why they couldn't enjoy a splash in an inviting pool in the hot African sun.

An elderly Iramba woman came to the hospital clinic because of an eye infection. After she had been given ointment for that complaint, she indicated another problem saying in Swahili, "Pia nina nyoka tumboni." (Also, I have a snake in my belly). She indicated that she had lost weight in spite of being very hungry and eating more than usual over the past few months. She occasionally had diarrhea and had seen some flat white structures in her stools. She brought us a sample which proved to be a section of a beef tapeworm. Each one-half-inch segment contains both male and female reproductive organs and produces about 80,000 fertile microscopic eggs. Her blood smear showed a large number of eosinophiles, white blood cells which are characteristic of parasitic infections. She admitted that she liked to eat beef which had been prepared by charring briefly over an open fire. She appeared healthy except for a prominent abdomen which was out of proportion for the rest of her physique.

We treated her with atabrine and gave her a cathartic. She passed a tapeworm which was at least twenty-six feet long and filled a one quart jar. It appeared somewhat like (Please pardon the analogy!) a long segmented string of egg noodles. We were pleased to see that it included the head section. Had the head not been passed, new body segments would have continued developing and she would have needed repeat treatment.

An American mother told me about a tapeworm experience with her five-year-old son. He spent much time with African playmates and their families. After she found the tell-tale worm segments in his stools, he was treated successfully. She was horrified at the size of the creature which he passed.

We saw many patients at Kiomboi and Iambi with beef tapeworm. The soil becomes contaminated through the careless deposit of waste by infected humans. Cattle ingest the eggs while grazing, and larvae develop in their tissue. Proper disposal of human waste and thorough cooking of meat effectively prevents the spread of tapeworm.

An estimated 40 percent of the people in the world harbor one or more species of worms. Most victims live in the developing countries of the tropics and subtropics. A certain percentage of us who live in the relatively worm-free world may pay a price. During my years in Africa I was surprised at how few allergies we seemed to encounter in our African patients. In America about one out of every five patients of all races in a doctor's office has hay fever, pollen or dust-triggered asthma, skin rashes, intolerance to animal's hair, or some other obviously allergic disorder. In Tanganyika I rarely saw people with any of these problems. Of course, we had more than enough disease to keep us busy so I was pleased not to have to deal with a lot of sneezes, wheezes, and itches. When we returned to America, I asked allergists about my observations and they didn't seem to believe me. One of them said that I was too busy with all those tropical diseases to notice the allergies.

I was intrigued to read an article in the September 1993 Discover Magazine by Dr. Eric Otteson, an allergist who is also the head of Parasitology at The National Institute of Allergy and Infectious Diseases in Bethesda, Maryland. He is convinced that people with certain parasitic disorders have far fewer allergic problems. Nineteen years earlier he had been involved with a project to treat the natives of Mauke in the Cook Islands, for filariasis. This disease is caused by mosquito-borne larvae, thread-like worms, which invade the lymphatic tissue and results in horrible swelling and disfigurement of the legs, genitals and breasts. It is known as elephantiasis. Thirty-five per cent of the population harbored the parasites. They were all treated in 1971. In 1992 Dr. Otteson returned with a team of specialists to study the health of all 600 people on the island. He found that the incidence of filariasis was way down, but that the percentage of people with allergies had increased dramatically from 3 percent to over 15 percent. The Number One offender was a severe form of octopus allergy which had been unknown two decades earlier. Many other inhabitants of the island were miserable for the first time with all the nasty symptoms of allergies.

Dr. Otteson and others are accumulating evidence that the presence of internal parasites appear to mute or reduce the allergic reaction to other substances. Wouldn't it be interesting if, at some time in the future, doctors learn how to treat their patients by infecting them with a few harmless pet worms to prevent some of the coughing, wheezing, sneezing, swelling and itching caused by allergies? When some of my doctor friends read this they are going to say, "John's been out in the tropical sun too much without wearing his pith helmet!"

21. "HER BLOOD CELLS LOOK LIKE THE NEW MOON!"

One sunny afternoon at Kiomboi Hospital, our African pastor, Manase Yona, knocked on my office door. Accompanied by his wife, he carried his seriously ill daughter, Joyce, into my office. With tears in his eyes, this kind, caring father gently laid her on my examining table. She was writhing in pain with her knees drawn up to her abdomen. When I carefully felt her tummy, the muscles were as rigid as a board. My first impression was appendicitis, but I was informed that her appendix had been removed two years earlier. In fact, there were two long surgical scars on her abdomen. The hospital records showed that she had first been operated upon for suspected appendicitis, and a few months later, for possible intestinal obstruction.

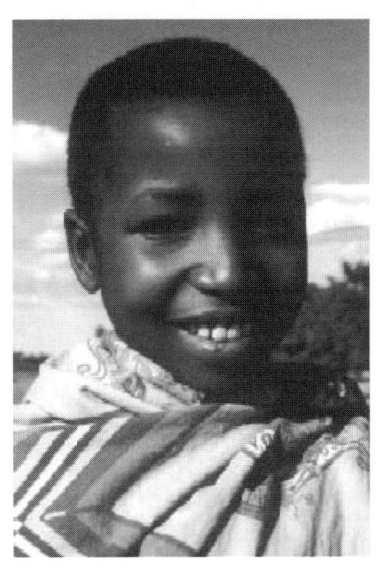

Joyce Manase

Joyce complained of severe pain in her abdomen, hands, and feet. The parents indicated that she had had many similar episodes of pain. During these attacks, which lasted several days, she became extremely weak and pale. Even when she was relatively well, there was much pain in her stomach and extremities.

Before she had been brought into my office, Yakobo, an experienced dresser, had already done a routine blood smear to check for malaria. Although he had limited formal education, he had become proficient in the use of the microscope in identifying malaria and a variety of parasitic disorders. Excitedly he came to me, saying, "There's something strange about Joyce's blood smear! Many of her red cells have the shape of the new moon!" When I focused the microscope, it was clear that he had made an astute observation. Instead of a normal donut shape, most of the red cells had assumed an elongated crescent shape. They did look like new moons or sickles. Aha! This little girl almost certainly had sickle cell anemia. I had been told that this disease hadn't been seen at Kiomboi. My predecessor, who had twice operated on Joyce, had trained many years earlier at a medical school with a limited number of Afro-American patients. In those days few doctors in America or Europe were aware of sickle cell anemia.

With what Yakobo and I had seen with the microscope, plus all of her symptoms and a hemoglobin less than 50 percent of normal, there was no doubt in my mind that she was a victim of this horrible affliction. I shuddered when I thought of what she and her family had been through and what was probably yet to come. (A few years earlier in America, a Negro mother had informed me with intense feeling, "My son has sick-as-hell anemia!" And that was an appropriate description.) We hospitalized Joyce and gave her fluids to correct the dehydration and acidosis which had triggered this sickle cell crisis. The term crisis is used to identify an episode in which there is massive destruction of red blood cells accompanied by an increase in pain and weakness. If the crisis is severe, death may follow. Some patients die of overwhelming infections probably related to poor circulation and impaired immune responses.

Research indicates that 12-15 percent of American Negroes are carriers of a single sickle cell gene. It is the most common lethal gene of humans. Approximately one of every 350 members of this population inherit the gene from both parents and are afflicted with full-blown sickle cell anemia. Even with optimum medical care they may not live to adulthood. Some authorities believed that in rural Africa most children with this disease died before their second birthday.

Nearly all of the hemoglobin of those with the disease is of the abnormal S type. Those with the carrier state, or sickle cell trait, have about 40 percent of hemoglobin of this type which is not enough to result in major health problems. Under conditions of lowered blood oxygen, acidosis, or dehydration, the abnormal S hemoglobin of patients with sickle cell anemia congeals into long crystals or fibers which distort the shape of the red cells and eventually cause them to rupture. The abnormally shaped cells do not flow normally through tiny blood vessels. They produce obstructive logjams especially in the capillaries of the spleen, fingers, toes and intestinal tract. This accounts for a part of the severe pain during a sickle cell crisis.

We are indebted to Nobel Prize winning chemist Linus Pauling for determining the exact chemical nature of the disease. He discovered that there was a difference of only one simple amino acid between normal adult hemoglobin and that of sickle cell disease. More recently scientists have determined the exact location and structure of the abnormal gene. Researchers speculate on the possibility of replacing the defective gene through new technology currently being developed in the field of genetic engineering.

Forty years ago an intriguing paradox arose when it was discovered that children with sickle cell trait had a higher than expected survival rate from the most virulent form of malaria which kills over a million African children every year. The parasites do not thrive in the cells which contain 40% S hemoglobin. Virtually all people with this abnormal hemoglobin originated in geographic areas in which this species of malaria existed. This included not only the Negro population, but a smaller percentage of people from Mediterranean countries, the Middle-east, and the Indian subcontinent. Here was a lethal gene which in the carrier state provides a significant survival advantage, and seems to have originated exactly where this vicious malaria species also prevails.

Over several days in the hospital, Joyce gradually improved. After discharge, her hemoglobin remained about half what it should have been; she had continuous aches and pains, and had to be hospitalized on numerous other occasions. Her parents patiently nurtured and comforted her in every possible way. I admired and respected them as beautiful human beings. Joyce herself was a model patient, suffering in silence until the symptoms abated.

I was eager to determine the approximate incidence of the sickle cell gene in our Iramba population. We had only a simple crude method to investigate the problem. A drop of blood was placed between two layers of glass and sealed around the edges with vaseline. As the oxygen is consumed by the trapped cells, S hemoglobin congeals and causes the cells to sickle in a matter of hours. This can be observed under the microscope and indicates the trait or carrier state.

First I checked Pastor Manase and his family. Both parents were strongly positive, as well as two of their four children. Their youngest child Benjamin had died a year earlier from measles at the age of fifteen months. The mother was convinced that he had the same symptoms as Joyce. It's quite probable that he also had sickle cell anemia. I showed Pastor Manase the abnormal cells under the microscope. He asked, "What does this mean if Joyce has children?" I explained that it might be difficult for her to have babies, but that if she married somebody just like herself all of her children would have the disease. If she married a man with the carrier state, about half of her children would be sick like herself. He responded, "I'll see that she doesn't marry anybody who has this condition." I was certain that if Joyce were to live to have serious suitors, Pastor Manase would see that they 'passed' the blood test.

During the next few months we randomly checked over five hundred Iramba patients as they came to the clinic. I found that 14 percent showed definite sickling, close to the average of the American Negro population. In a couple of instances, I found the trait in husband and wife. Each of these couples had had children die before the age of two with stories suggestive of sickle cell anemia. I saw only one other living person with the full-blown disease, a three-year-old, whose mother brought him in because of pain and swelling of the fingers.

After we returned to the States, I received several letters from Pastor Manase wondering if there was anything new to help poor Joyce. The following is a translation from the one of his Swahili letters written in 1969:

"With this letter I wish to let you know of the health problems of our daughter Joyce. I believe you will remember her because you are the one who discovered that she had sickle cell anemia. She is now seventeen years old but continues having terrible attacks about every two months but often even more frequently than that. She has awful pain in her arms, legs, chest, and stomach. It grieves us to hear her cries for relief for the next ten days or more. When the pain subsides, she feels relatively well. We pray that the next episode will never come but it always does. Please let us know if there is any new treatment which might help Joyce!"

Unfortunately, I had to reply that there had been no significant breakthroughs in the therapy of sickle cell anemia. Joyce's health slowly deteriorated and she died a painful death in her early twenties.

At this time there is still no specific treatment available. Progress has been made in shortening the attacks, relieving pain, and preventing infection. Sickle cell anemia can be prevented by seeing that carriers do not have children by other carriers or by persons who have the full-blown disease. I hope that in the coming years a complete cure will be developed so that fewer and fewer children like Joyce will have to suffer as she did.

22. MEDICAL EXAMINER FOR HER MAJESTY'S COURT

Tanganyika was an outpost of the British Empire. The judicial and penal systems were administered by colonial officers who were directly under the top hierarchy in London. Since we missionary doctors were often the only physicians in remote areas, we were deputized to perform certain medicolegal functions for the local government. This included examination of prisoners, autopsies in the case of violent or unexplained deaths, and other coroner-type responsibilities. Every time I received a subpoena or directive with Her Majesty's elegant letterhead at the top, I felt that young Queen Elizabeth was sending a personal message to me.

Corporal punishment was still one of the options of the penal code used primarily on young prisoners who had committed minor offenses, such as theft. I heard our African District Commissioner defend this mode of discipline as being both humane and more effective than incarceration. Being jailed for a few days with free room and board was not as likely to deter repeat offenses as a sore bottom and a little humiliation. No, I didn't do the caning myself, but it was my responsibility to examine the prisoner before it was accomplished. A policeman would bring the young offender to my office with an affidavit to be signed indicating that there was no underlying medical condition which would contraindicate a certain number of strokes of the cane.

The dimensions of said implement were strictly prescribed. It was a flexible wooden wand, about two and a half feet long, tapered from a diameter of one half-inch at the thick end down to less than one-quarter inch at the other. After I examined the young miscreant and affixed my signature to Her Majesty's official document, he was lead back to headquarters for implementation of the sentence. Usually it consisted of ten to fifteen strokes of the cane which were administered by an African policeman in the presence of a senior member of the staff. In none of the six young prisoners who were brought to me over the years did I find anything which would rule out the punishment.

I did have mixed emotions about the whole thing. Among other things, I wondered if I would be liable if one of these fellows should die during the caning. Actually, the severity of the spanking was probably comparable to that which my father had inflicted on me five or six times in my youthful days for major offenses. The only difference was that my dad, with tears in his eyes, would later take me in his arms, tell me why he had punished me and indicate how much he loved me.

The young Tanganyikans didn't receive that part of the treatment from Her Majesty.

In medical school I had done well in the subject of pathology, ranking fifth in my class. Our professor, who was also dean of the medical school, suggested that I should consider a career in pathology. I told him that I enjoyed people too much to be attracted to a life in the morgue and the laboratory. Ten years later in Africa, I was to become an instant pathologist. I had assisted with several autopsies as a medical student but had never done one alone. The local police would soon see that I had that privilege. About twice a month the Kiomboi constabulary would bring us a body and say, "Okay Doc, you tell us what caused this death."

We had a complete set of post-mortem surgical instruments, and I got well acquainted with all of them. A common cause of death was ruptured spleens with massive internal bleeding. Most of the local population had enlarged fragile spleens from chronic malaria. A slight blow to the left upper abdomen could rupture them. Ruptured tubal pregnancies also took a toll. If the cause of death was clear, we were not required to do a complete autopsy but, by doing so, we often gained valuable information about the health of the population. For example, I was amazed at how healthy the coronary arteries of elderly Africans appeared in comparison with those of Americans of the same age. If the answer was not forthcoming from our examination, we sent tissue specimens to the pathologist in Dar es Salaam. It took over a month to receive an answer.

One morning near the end of the rainy season, two African policemen drove up to the hospital in a Land Rover. They presented me with a post-mortem requisition, but no corpse. I was asked to bring my instruments and accompany them.

Our destination was a village about thirty miles away where a young woman had disappeared under mysterious circumstances. In the hot mid-day sun we drove down the Rift Valley escarpment onto the Wembere Plains over a bumpy, barely visible road. As we neared our destination, we were engulfed by dark rain-clouds and drenched by a brief torrential downpour. We could drive no farther so we waded a flooded gully and walked the last mile to a small village. One of the policemen carried the heavy case containing my instruments. At the village we were met by the local chief and the parents of the missing woman. They gave the following story:

The young woman had been married a year earlier as the second wife of a man with a good reputation. He had paid the agreed-upon bride price to the father and all seemed in order. She moved into her husband's home after the wedding but returned to visit her parents in a nearby village about once a month. When she hadn't visited them for several weeks, they went to investigate. Next-door neighbors hadn't seen her but assumed that she had returned to her parents' home. Her co-wife at first denied that anything was amiss. Under intense questioning, she broke down and cried. She then admitted that the husband had struck the young woman with his fist when she talked back to him. He hadn't hit her hard, but still she keeled over and died. He pledged the first wife to secrecy under threat of violence. They buried the body under the floor of their hut, but a week later on a dark night, they moved it to a deeper grave in a sweet potato patch one hundred yards away. After this confession, the local chief arrested the husband and sent him off to jail. The family was ordered not to disturb the grave until the police investigation was complete.

Relatives had maintained a twenty-four-hour vigil at the burial site except when they were chased away by a herd of elephants who wanted to sample the sweet potatoes. When we arrived, the entire clan was clustered around the grave. We requested that the remains be carefully exhumed. The body had been wrapped in several layers of cowhide and buried about four feet deep. I gingerly unwrapped the month-old corpse and proceeded with my investigation. This included an examination of the brain, which is difficult even under ideal conditions. I found no evidence of broken bones or internal bleeding so my final report was inconclusive. We never received information about the outcome of this case.

On only one occasion was I subpoenaed to testify in court. I had performed an autopsy on the body of an elderly Iramba woman. She had been savagely beaten to death with a heavy wooden club by a man who was convinced that she had bewitched his young son, causing him to have a high fever. The child was taken to the clinic and treated for malaria from which he rapidly recovered.

My examination of the corpse revealed fractures of every major bone of the arms and legs. At the trial the judge and chief prosecutor were British and the defense lawyer was East Indian. All three wore the traditional long white curly wigs. Under oath, I gave my testimony describing the injuries. In his defense, the accused stated his absolute conviction that he was saving his son by attacking the witch. He had never been in trouble with the law before. He was sentenced to be hanged. My feeling of sympathy included him as well as the victim and her family. He too became a victim of the powerful and pervasive persuasions of his culture.

My most heart-wrenching experience as a medical examiner occurred not long before we returned to America. A tall sad-faced African policeman led a young woman into my office carrying a small bundle wrapped in bloodstained yellow muslin. Utter desolation and grief was etched in her face, yet there was also a Madonna-like serenity and composure. She was carrying all that remained of her eight-year-old daughter wrapped in a fragment of her dress. When the little girl had failed to return from school the preceding afternoon, she was thought to be with friends or visiting her grandmother. By sunset the family became alarmed and a torchlight search was mounted. Not until the next morning did they find the place where hyenas had caught the little girl. My responsibility was to identify and describe the few fragments of bone from the skull, shoulder blade and pelvis.

After I had finished, the grief-stricken mother carefully re-wrapped the pathetic little bundle. She then turned toward me with a sad brief smile and a barely audible farewell and walked slowly out of the room. As I wrote my report to police headquarters, I found myself struggling to maintain my own composure. My heart went out to all of the mothers and fathers who had suffered the loss of a child under any circumstances, but especially such tragedy as this poor mother endured.

23. "THERE'S A LEOPARD IN MY HOUSE!"

Most of my experiences with dangerous animals were second hand. I patched up over thirty people who had been attacked by leopards, lions, hyenas, rhinos, and elephants. None of the attacking predators were man-eaters. They had learned that domestic livestock were much easier to catch than wild game. While we were in Tanganyika, one man-eating lion did kill and devour seven people in a community about sixty miles from Kiomboi. When the game department finally destroyed this animal, they found he was an ancient male who had porcupine quills in his paws and was no longer able to catch his natural prey.

Most of the people I sewed up had been mauled by leopards in or near their homes. At Kiomboi Hospital, a middle-aged Iramba man came to my office with his right hand wrapped in a frayed old bandage. Under this tattered covering, we found a badly scarred hand with contraction and stiffening of the fingers.

How had this serious damage occurred? One night a leopard had jumped through a window into his neighbor's house. The entire family rushed out the door and shut it behind them. Only then did they realize they had left the three-year-old daughter asleep in her bed. With the leopard snarling at the door, no one volunteered to go in to get the child who by this time was screaming in terror.

A missionary who lived nearby was called. Hurrying to the site with his rifle, he found a wildly chaotic scene with much noise and confusion. A brief council led to an attempt to rescue the little girl through a hole made in the wall near her bed by chiseling out one of the 8 x 12-inch mud bricks. Our hero put his arm through the opening in an effort to reach the child. Unfortunately, he inserted his hand directly into the mouth of the waiting leopard. With a mighty effort, he succeeded in pulling the big cat's head out far enough so that the missionary could safely shoot it. The little girl was unharmed but her would-be-rescuer's hand was badly chewed up.

This injury, complicated by a serious infection, resulted in a disability. He somehow came to the conclusion that, since we Americans were involved in this episode, it behooved us to pay him workman's compensation. We had no budgets for such contingencies. With exercises and a bit of simple physiotherapy, he gradually regained most of the function he had lost.

Another patient at Kiomboi was an old man who had been attacked by a leopard. He had been defending his livestock with his spear when the animal turned on him. With a vicious swipe, the angry cat literally ripped off his scalp. An area of the skull five inches in diameter was exposed. This tough old guy survived the bleeding and shock and was brought to the hospital. Unfortunately, the missing scalp wasn't retrieved so it was impossible to close the huge skin defect.

A month later growth around the edges had made the exposed area of skull only slightly smaller. I was the only doctor at the time and was not skilled enough in plastic surgery to cover this huge defect using skin flaps. Dr. Moris at Iambi suggested an almost medieval technique which he had observed in China to grow skin over the exposed bone. A series of holes ¼-inch in diameter is drilled just through the outer layer of the exposed skull in a grid pattern about ½-inch apart. In an effort to heal these holes, live tissue grows up from the marrow cavity and literally creates a carpet of so-called proud flesh over the bone. I thought that the risk of leaving his bone exposed to the outside world was greater than the danger of this unorthodox procedure. With the patient anesthetized, I took a bone drill and carefully drilled rows of holes. When I finished, the top of his skull looked something like a miniature Chinese checkerboard.

It worked! Six weeks later, all of the exposed bone was covered by a pink layer of living tissue. I was then able to graft strips of skin from his legs. Eventually, when the whole area was resurfaced with a layer of skin, the old gentleman was quite proud of his new dome. A cute little fringe of hair grew around a rough pink bald pate. It wasn't very pretty, but reminded me of the hair style of the Benedictine monks in the 16th century. The delicate skin badly needed protection from the bright sun so we gave him an old cap which he wore at a jaunty angle.

The last time I saw him, he was seated in the midst of a cluster of people under a big fig tree outside the hospital. He was gesturing vigorously with his hands probably telling them all about his adventures. Then he ceremoniously doffed his cap to show everybody what the leopard and that crazy doctor from America had done to the top of his head.

One day I was called to the hospital to see a woman with leprosy who had been attacked by a rhino. She had been walking down a trail in thick bushy terrain when she encountered the animal face to face. When he charged, his huge horn went directly into her mouth, tearing it from ear to ear. She remained conscious until she had been carried to the hospital. I was able to repair her mouth but there were fractures of the bones of the base of her skull with leakage of spinal fluid. Three days later she died of meningitis in spite of large doses of antibiotics.

Then there was the man who was stepped on by an elephant and lived to tell about it. He had been hoeing in his cornfield when the elephant walked up behind him, picked him up with his trunk, tossed him high in the air, and then stepped on him. His horrified young wife witnessed the entire episode and was sure that she had just become a widow.

After the elephant went on his way, the trembling woman was vastly relieved when she heard a cry for help from her husband. The family quickly rescued him and brought him to the hospital. My examination showed that the elephant had stepped on both thighs but the weight went between them so that no bones were broken. There was extensive crushing injury of the muscles, but in time the man was able to walk with only a slight limp.

In 1958 I cared for a young Barabaig warrior who had been mauled by a lion. He and about fifteen of his fellow morani went after the animal which had killed one of their cattle.

When they surrounded the creature in thick brush, he volunteered to go in and scare it out. The lioness sprang upon him, badly mangling his left shoulder and upper arm before the other morani could come to his rescue and dispatch the lion.

He was carried several miles to our hospital two days later. I was horrified to see how much damage a lion's jaw could inflict on the tissue of a strong young man. By this time the wounds were seriously infected, and we nearly lost our patient in spite of vigorous antibiotic treatment. After recovery, his left shoulder was permanently disabled. He was awarded the lion skin since he had drawn first blood. In recognition of his bravery, he became an elite and respected elder in his tribe.

The episode of repairing animal-inflicted damage which I remember most vividly began in the middle of a night illuminated by a gorgeous full moon. I was awakened from a deep sleep by a loud knocking on our bedroom window and a excited voice calling, "Hodi! Hodi!" Two African nurses, one carrying a lantern, excitedly told me that there was a serious emergency. I quickly dressed and ran the quarter of a mile to the hospital.

In our emergency room I found an anguished group of people clustered around a man holding a child covered with blood from head to toe. This little fellow, about ten years old, had been attacked by a leopard which had entered the house intent on stealing a lamb or goat. The father had come to the rescue with his spear, wounding the big cat and causing him to flee out the window.

The boy was obviously in pain but didn't let out a whimper. He looked up at me with big trusting eyes which melted my heart. Most of the bleeding had stopped, but his body was covered with gaping wounds from the left side of his face down to his lower legs. His blood pressure and heart rate were normal so he was not in physical shock. As I gently cleaned his injuries, he flinched and silently gritted his teeth. He looked up at me and calmly answered my questions. Under Novocain anesthesia, I sewed up his ugly wounds, putting in over two hundred stitches. After I had put the last one in place and bandaged him from head to ankle, he smiled shyly, wordlessly but eloquently expressing his thanks. As we carried him to his hospital bed, a spectacular sunrise lit up the eastern horizon. His night of horror was over and a new day had begun.

24. ANIMAL DOCTOR

In preparing to work in Tanganyika, one of the responsibilities I hadn't anticipated was dealing with the medical problems of the animal population. I soon discovered that, in the absence of veterinarians, the Africans expected me to treat their ailing livestock. One of the Iramba elders put it this way, "If your medicine is good for people, surely it will help our animals!"

Aside from their economic value, cattle, donkeys, goats and chickens were very much a part of an Iramba household. They had to be protected from lions, hyenas and leopards especially at night. At dusk domestic animals were brought inside the courtyard adjacent to the family quarters until morning. Often a separate room was attached to the house for the smaller, more vulnerable animals. Any disturbance at night was immediately checked out. Men and older boys defended their livestock with spears and clubs, often sustaining terrible injuries.

Even small children played a role in the care and protection of the animals. Once while out walking near Iambi, we came upon a little boy not more than six years of age herding a small group of lambs. He was armed with a big knobkerrie club. When I asked him what he was doing, he brandished his big stick and proudly announced, "Ninafukuza nyani!" (I am chasing away the baboons!) These wily primates are definitely a threat to small animals. With this degree of investment in the care and protection of their creatures, it wasn't surprising that they would expect their doctor to play his part as well.

My initial therapeutic success at Iambi involved a sick dog. Every one of my first five human patients had died. These included a man with an appendix which had been ruptured for several days, an ancient woman mauled by a hyena, and a young mother with a ruptured uterus. I wondered if any of my patients would ever survive.

Then Stan Alderson, the British superintendent of construction of our new leprosy facility, asked me to take a look at his ailing mutt. Simba (Swahili for lion) was an astounding specimen. Allegedly his mother was a Rhodesian Ridgeback and his father, a Dachshund. Ridgebacks are huge dogs, weighing close to one hundred pounds, especially bred to hunt leopards. We wondered how this mismatch had been accomplished. Simba weighed over sixty pounds with a long sausage-shaped body and stubby legs which barely kept his belly off the ground. He was the ugliest dog I had ever seen, but much loved by seven-year-old Jane and five-year-old Michael Alderson. They were devastated when Simba became feverish, stopped eating, and appeared to be dying. When I examined him, he gazed sorrowfully up at me and weakly wagged his tail. I discovered a large abscess around the liver.

After surgically draining this, I injected him with generous doses of penicillin and streptomycin. I didn't really expect him to survive, but by the next morning he was already up and eating. Within a week he was waddling happily around playing with Michael and Jane. After this breakthrough, I began having reassuring successes with my human patients, too.

One Sunday morning, as I was preparing to go to church, an Iramba farmer appeared at the back door leading a cow. She had delivered a calf the day before but hadn't passed the afterbirth. In human mothers a retained placenta represents a serious problem, so I assumed that it was important to do something for this poor creature. Since the animal seemed to be in good shape, I told the man to return at noon.

After worshipping at church and seeing my human patients in the hospital, I picked up a pair of arm-length rubber gloves and prepared to help my bovine patient. She was laid on the ground and her legs were restrained by several pairs of strong arms. From an almost prone position, I went to work. I was able to remove the reluctant placenta with great difficulty. It would have been easier if I had been equipped with a smaller right hand. The patient recovered uneventfully. Unfortunately, word of my success got around so I was asked to repeat the performance on several subsequent occasions.

At Iambi in 1958 I was the only doctor for both the hospital and the leprosy program. We had been assured that the region, previously unoccupied, was free of tsetse flies, and therefore suitable for cattle. In order to make the colony more self-sufficient, our agriculturist, Roly Renner, purchased a herd of forty cattle. These were cared for by some of the least-disabled leprosy patients.

A month later some of the animals became sick and two died. We made a tour of the area in which they had been grazing and found tsetse flies. I should say that they found us for we were bitten several times. They aggressively attack any warm-blooded creature including man. Their tough beetle-like bodies make them difficult to kill with a fly swatter or with a mere slap of the hand. (Dan called them taxi flies.) Fortunately for us, they carried only animal trypanosomiasis and not the dreaded African sleeping sickness which claims so many human lives in other parts of Africa.

On the other hand, our cattle were in big trouble! If we didn't do something soon we would lose them all. We dispatched an urgent telegram to the animal husbandry division in Dar es Salaam. Within a week we received a supply of the medicine to be given to the sick cattle. Accompanying instructions indicated the amount to be given by injection. Since we had no veterinary equipment, I had to borrow from the hospital. Our largest needles, 18-guage, were not adequate to puncture tough cowhide, but we had to make do.

With our paraphernalia, we entered the arena, a log corral with the big Brahma-like cattle milling about. The situation had all the makings of a real Wild West rodeo complete with an excited crowd of patients cheering us on from the top rails. The restless animals weren't particularly interested in submitting to treatment by a pale-faced quack horse-doctor.

We had no restraining chutes but one of the patients, who had badly deformed feet and only stumps of fingers, was quite skillful with a lasso. He didn't go for the head and horns but, after a merry chase, managed somehow to get his rope around one of the front legs. Then about ten other men with varying degrees of deformity would grab the rope. After a few mad circuits around the corral, they managed to stop and partially immobilize their victim. They would yell at me in Swahili, "Okay Doc! Do your thing!" As soon as I approached, the animal would make a few more turns around the arena. I would then sneak up as close as possible and make a wild stab at the closest part of the anatomy. As often as not, the needle would break off or bend double and we'd start all over again. At one point the herd bull lunged at me as I was standing in front of a tree in the middle of the corral. I sidestepped quickly, and he hit the tree with a mighty thud, nearly knocking himself out.

After each animal was treated, it was escorted out of the enclosure. The last one took the longest time because there was more running room. In some ways the ordeal reminded me of some of the tussles I had experienced with reluctant children in examining rooms back in the States. After the operation was completed in two hours, a round of applause arose from the assembled crowd. Only one more animal died. We were able to pasture the herd in a portion of the range which was free of tsetse flies.

There were other adventures in amateur veterinary medicine. Several times I had to draw the line and indicate that certain animal health problems were beyond my professional competence. One such occasion arose with the urgent request of our African pastor to examine his donkey which had accidentally stepped into a warthog hole. I found the poor creature gingerly standing on three legs with the right rear extremity skewed at a grotesque angle because of a broken femur. His owner wondered if I couldn't put on a cast like we did for humans with broken bones. I indicated that this would be very difficult since no weight could be born on that leg. Poor old Punda would have had a tough time using crutches!

Another episode involved a cow which had been in labor for two days. After we had spent an hour trying to extract the already-dead calf, I made the suggestion that perhaps it would be best for them to take this suffering animal home and let her make the ultimate sacrifice to provide a feast for the clan. That's just what they did.

I thoroughly enjoy animals, both domestic and wild, but back here in America I am quite content to leave their health problems in the competent hands of a friendly veterinarian!

25. "HOW COULD YOU SHOOT THAT BEAUTIFUL CREATURE?"

Before going to Africa I had never owned a firearm. My only experience with rifles came in infantry basic training in Texas during World War II. I passed the marksmanship course on the firing range with an M1 rifle, but certainly didn't distinguish myself. In Tanganyika there was a special incentive to become more familiar with guns. If we were to have any meat other than the stringy beef butchered locally, it would be up to me to provide it.

My first opportunity to experience a hunting safari came a month after our arrival. Rev. Bob Ward was a skilled and experienced hunter. He took part of his vacation time to escort a party of four American doctors into the game-rich Yaida Valley in quest of elephant and Cape buffalo trophies. I was supposed to be diligently studying Swahili during those first six weeks, but I jumped at an opportunity to rendezvous with the hunting party already out in the bush. I rationalized that I could learn the language there, too.

One of our doctors, Leonard Linnell, and his wife Claire, had planned a one day trip to the hunting camp to see their American friends. They invited me to accompany them. I grabbed my pith helmet, a friend's double-barreled shotgun, my cameras, and a canteen of water. I kissed Adeline goodbye and assured her that I would be back by nightfall. In spite of my good intentions, she would not see me again for four days.

I hopped into the jeep with Len, Claire, and an African guide and off we drove! For four hours we bounced over a barely discernible road through ruggedly beautiful countryside. We finally arrived at the riverside acacia-grove where the hunting party was supposed to be camped, but they weren't at our rendezvous site.

Since we had been invited to have lunch with the hunters, we hadn't brought any food. By mid-afternoon we were mighty hungry. In a nearby ravine we heard the cackling of a flock of guinea fowl. I grabbed the shotgun, loaded it, and crept cautiously until I was near enough to see my quarry. At least a dozen birds were busily feeding within forty feet of me. Knowing that I couldn't possibly hit them in flight, I fired both barrels into their midst while they were innocently having dinner. Six of them fluttered helplessly on the ground. They were the first creatures I had ever dispatched with a gun and I didn't feel particularly good about it. I felt like a mass murderer. I was less remorseful after we had cleaned, spitted and roasted a couple of young birds on the coals of our open fire. The meat was tender and delicious.

Late in the afternoon the hunting party finally arrived, having been delayed by mechanical problems on one of their vehicles. After they had set up camp under a large fig tree, we enjoyed a robust meal, enlivened by stories of the day's hunting adventures. Among other feats, they had shot two elephants.

Dr. Linnell had to return to the hospital so I reluctantly prepared to leave with him. Bob Ward suggested that I stay with them for the last three days of the safari. He didn't need to twist my arm. I could study Swahili any time, but when would I get another opportunity like this. Bob found an extra sleeping bag and shared his tent with me. When I lay down and closed my eyes, all I could see were guinea fowl flopping helplessly on the ground. We went to sleep to the night music of distant lions and nearby hyenas and were awakened by a melodious symphony of bird songs.

Those next three days comprised an exciting introduction to the African bush. On the first morning Bob and the African guide led us several miles through dense underbrush on the trail of a large buffalo. Suddenly Mr. Buffalo charged out of the trees directly toward us. Five rifles, none smaller than .375 caliber, emitted a mighty barrage. The huge animal finally went down not twenty feet from the tree behind which I was hiding with my movie camera. Did I capture this dramatic episode on film? I'm afraid not; I was too busy fleeing to cover. For years this magnificent buffalo head, with its massive horns, was mounted on the wall of the downtown hardware store in Worthington, Minnesota.

Many other adventures were packed into those three days in the Yaida Valley. While on a solo stroll near our camp, I was thrilled to come upon a pair of African wild hunting dogs as they emerged from their den. The moment they saw me they barked and scampered back underground. They were the only wild dogs i saw in Africa.

I particularly enjoyed getting acquainted with young Marko and Mickey Bicchieri, sons of an Italian gold miner who operated a mine near Kiomboi. They were co-leaders of the expedition with Bob. Marko was interested in pursuing a medical career. He and I did some serious anatomical dissection while cleaning an impala shot by one of the hunters. Marko eventually became a distinguished professor of anthropology at a university in Washington. Mickey settled in northern British Columbia as a gold miner and logger. We had a happy reunion with him and his wife many years later on a trip to Alaska.

Those four days of introduction to the African bush slipped by all too rapidly. We headed back to Isanzu with the vehicles heavily loaded with trophies and meat. Of necessity, I had lived in the same set of clothes twenty-four hours a day. When we finally arrived home, my family was glad to see me but they didn't get very close until I had bathed.

Game was abundant within a few miles of our home but first I had to acquire a weapon. I soon had the opportunity to purchase a 9.3 mm Mauser rifle which had been brought to Africa many years earlier. With its hexagonal barrel and well-worn stock it appeared ancient but was in excellent condition. Ammunition for this odd caliber firearm came from Czechoslovakia. After a session of target practice, I was ready to feed my family.

All the meat on our table for the next three years was provided by my trusty Mauser. On the first hunt, I fired only two bullets which brought down an impala and a hartebeest. Our African guides were impressed, but they subsequently discovered that the Bwana Daktari Yohana had just experienced some beginner's luck.

Approximately every six weeks I broke away from the hospital to restock our larder. Our little kerosene refrigerator had only a small freezing compartment so Adeline often canned the surplus meat. Our favorite flavors were eland, wildebeest, impala, and hartebeest. If nothing else was available, I would sometimes bring home a zebra. With the fat removed, Adeline ground the meat into fairly decent zebraburger. On one occasion we entertained the British Provincial Commissioner, who was inspecting our leprosy colony. The only meat available was ground zebra which Adeline cooked up into a savory hot dish. Our distinguished guest, whose counterpart in America would have been the governor of a state, enjoyed the meat well enough to ask for second and third helpings. We didn't tell him what he was eating!

On each hunting trip, I was accompanied by two or three Africans. They vied for the opportunity because it usually meant a share of meat for their cooking pots. For me, their presence was vital. As outdoors-men, they were major leaguers and I was a rank amateur. I marveled at their tracking ability and their sense of orientation. In mid-day when the sun was directly overhead and we were hunting in terrain with no visible landmarks, I was completely lost. It was then that they would ask me, "Okay Bwana! Where did we leave the jeep?" Much to their amusement, I would usually point in the wrong direction. Those who were Muslims invariably dashed to a downed animal to perform a ritual bleeding. Otherwise, they could not partake of the meat. When I missed an easy shot they consoled me. The camaraderie which we developed made these outings a source of many happy memories for me. My companions seemed to enjoy themselves, too.

I wanted a zebra skin as a memento of our African days. On one outing, I spotted just the right specimen. He was standing with his head over the shoulder of a companion in a mutual grooming posture. I stepped out of the jeep and crawled to within a hundred yards. Taking careful aim at his shoulder, I fired. My target galloped away but the friend, whose head was over his shoulder, collapsed in a heap. When we approached, we found that he was indeed dead, but no bullet hole was visible. Had I frightened him to death? A companion lifted the head and discovered that my bullet had entered the left eye. "What a shot, Bwana!" he exclaimed. I didn't tell him that I had aimed at the other zebra. Actually I missed the zebra's shoulder on which I was sighting by less than a foot.

On my last African hunting safari, we drove out on the Wembere plains to get a wildebeest. In less than an hour, I brought down a nice fat young male. We loaded the animal into our jeep truck and headed back toward Kiomboi. We passed near a handsome trio of Thompson's gazelle bucks and my African friends begged me to shoot one for them. Reluctantly I stopped, stepped out, aimed and fired. Unfortunately, I wounded one and had to walk at least a half-mile to get close. He was lying helplessly, but with head erect. As I approached, he slowly turned and looked at me with his big innocent eyes. Much as I hated to do so, I had no recourse but to complete my mission. We returned home and were met by our nurse-midwife Greta Engberg. Tommies were her favorite African animals. When she saw one in the truck, she berated me soundly, "How could you shoot that beautiful innocent creature!" She really let me have it with both barrels, and I was thoroughly cowed.

That night I had a vivid dream in which I relived the entire hunt. As I neared the wounded gazelle, he again turned his head, but with one difference. He was wearing the horn-rimmed glasses and facial features of my friend Greta. That woke me up immediately.

Not long afterwards, Kiomboi School for missionary children had a Halloween party. Adeline made animal masks for our family: elephant, zebra and giraffe for the children and for me, a gazelle complete with real horns and glasses similar to Greta's. I planned to wear it to the party, carrying a huge book entitled; "All About People by T. Gazelle." Just as we were dressing up, I was called to the hospital to help Dr. Lofstrom with emergency surgery.

A middle-aged man had just been carried in because of a strangulated inguinal hernia. He had been suffering at home for a week and was going into shock. We had to remove a foot of gangrenous bowel. We were fearful that he wouldn't survive the operation. The next morning, we were amazed to find him bright and alert, asking when he could go home. A week later, he walked out of the hospital with a big smile on his face.

Of course, the Halloween party went on without me. Adeline wore the gazelle costume in my place, while Elly accompanied her wearing a hunting costume and carrying a wooden rifle. All the people at the party had heard the full story and my family made a big hit. Our best-laid plans were often thwarted by such unforeseen emergencies.

Since that sequence of the hunt, the scolding, and the dream I haven't fired at another animal except through the viewfinder of my camera.

26. "SIAFU! SIAFU!"

The billions of insects and other tiny creatures which bite, sting, infect, devour, and otherwise plague mankind, play leading roles in the lives of people in tropical Africa. Most of the time the bugs are cast as villains, but occasionally they prove themselves benevolent and beneficial. The following tales recount intimate personal encounters with crawlin' critters in Tanganyika.

The first night we slept in our new home at Iambi, we prepared for bed after a hectic day of unpacking and assembling furniture. Our oldest daughter Margaret was away in boarding school at Kiomboi so there were just the four of us at home. After hearing their bedtime prayers, we kissed Elly and Dan goodnight and tucked them under their mosquito nets. Adeline and I turned out our Coleman lantern, crawled into our own net-covered cocoon and settled down for the night.

As we were drifting off to sleep, we became aware of an eerie scratching sound from the corner of our bedroom. In the total darkness of the African night the "Scrape-Scrape-Scrape" seemed to grow louder and louder! What could it be? Our imaginations ran riot! We thought that mysterious noise most likely came from a rat or a snake. We couldn't sleep until we knew what was going on so I crawled out of bed, grabbed a flashlight, and turned it on. I focused the beam in the direction of the continuing sound, and it fell on a large cardboard packing box. When I cautiously peered into the empty carton, I discovered the largest bug I had ever seen. Fully three inches long, the huge black beetle was trying to crawl out of the box into which it had fallen. He couldn't get a grip on the side so kept falling back. I captured it in a glass jar for further study. Then we went to sleep with the less threatening sounds of a family of hyenas wailing, barking, and laughing in the distance. In the morning we identified the disturber of our slumber as one of a family of large nocturnal predator beetles. He was simply trying to rid our house of some of the other insects which might trouble us. After taking his picture, I released him in the great outdoors. Dr. Albert Schweitzer would have been proud of me!

We had many other encounters with nasty little creatures. A daily ritual on rising in the morning was shaking out one's shoes before putting them on. One day Elly shook out a three-inch centipede which could have given her a terribly painful bite. Other missionary friends had found scorpions hiding in their footwear. A sting by one of these is often fatal to a child under seven years of age. The stings of some species are more deadly than others but all are terribly painful. One of our mission doctors was stung on a finger by a scorpion and vividly described the excruciating pain. Injecting the site with Novocain gave no relief and the agony was only partially subdued by a shot of morphine.

On one occasion I was performing a surgical procedure in the operating room. We were startled to see a scorpion crawling down the I.V. tubing toward the patient. An African nurse flicked it off on the floor and dispatched it. How would that scenario play out if it transpired in a modern American surgery theater?

The most threatening and painful adventures with tiny creatures occurred early in our term. Soon after we went to sleep, we were awakened by screams from Dan's bedroom. Rushing to the rescue, we found that his room had been invaded by army ants, known in Swahili as siafu. A solid black wave of one-half to three-fourth-inch-long six-legged creatures was sweeping across one side of the room in a relentless tide. When they had reached Dan's bed, they climbed up one bedpost and found an opening through which they could crawl under the mosquito net. Dozens of them were swarming onto his arms, neck, and face, biting him unmercifully. From the opposite side of the bed, I was able to rescue him. As he continued screaming in terror and pain, we stripped off his pajamas and brushed away the ugly attackers. In doing so, Adeline and I received several painful bites. With their sharp pincers they latch securely onto the skin with a grip which persists even when their bodies are crushed.

At that moment, we saw a horde of ants crawling into Elly's room so we hastily rescued her before they reached her bed. Before our room was invaded, we placed the legs of the bed in pie tins filled with kerosene and tied an oil soaked rag around the hook in the ceiling from which our mosquito net was suspended. Then the four of us crowded into bed together. We discovered that we were more comfortable packed sardine-style with Mommy and Elly having their heads at the foot of the bed, with Dan and Daddy in the opposite direction.

Before we turned out the light, the marauders reached our room. We watched in fascination as the solid black wave slowly oozed through the door like thick syrup invading a pancake and spreading out to cover every square inch of the floor. Then, defying gravity, the invasive wave moved up the wall and across the ceiling. We were relieved that they were thwarted by our protective measures.

We turned out the lantern and slept fitfully. The bedcovers were pulled up and down and back and forth. Elly complained that Dan's feet were in her face. Somehow we survived the night but were happy to welcome the dawning of a new day.

By morning the invading army had gone on its way, and we thought we had escaped with only a few bites. Then we noticed that there were no sounds from the eight chickens in the little coop outside the kitchen door: the siafu had killed them all. Their limp bodies were scattered about suggesting that they had died in a desperate struggle.

Driver ants prey primarily on insects, but if other creatures are in their way they swarm into the respiratory passages and mouth, killing by suffocation. We heard stories of tiny babies being asphyxiated by ants. Even elephants are terrified by siafu. They do not actually dismember and eat their larger victims but seem to be attracted by the moisture of the respiratory passages.

When army ants return home in the morning from their night raids, they travel in serpentine columns. Some of them use their bodies to form a continuous enclosed geodesic archway by attaching themselves to each other. From above, this gives the appearance of a snake, scaring the birds which might otherwise feast on them. Through this tunnel the workers carry the booty of the night's raid, all manner of insect life. When the last of the workers pass through, the archway is dismantled and re-formed at the head of the line. I once measured a column which was over fifty yards long. If a moving colony is disturbed, thousands of soldier ants swarm to the defense and immediately repair the damaged archway.

They do not build their own nests. Sometimes they colonize a termite hill whose occupants they have killed and devoured. Here they live and raise their young while going on their raids. Naturalists have discovered that each foray radiates out in a different direction from their home base to cover a wedge of territory. The next raid sweeps through another segment, comparable to devouring a pie, a piece at a time from the center. When the pie is finished, the colony moves on to fresh territory.

Our home was invaded on five different nights during our first few months in Africa. Each time a different member of the family called out the alarm, "Siafu! Siafu!" Then we escaped to an un-invaded room of the house and established our lines of defense. In each instance we survived with only a few bites and were relieved to find that the marauding hordes had moved on before the next day dawned. After the third episode one of our veteran missionary friends wryly commented, "We are feeding our siafu a special diet this year-The Hults!"

27. COBRAS, PUFF ADDERS, PYTHONS, AND MAMBAS

Everyone who has spent more than a few days in East Africa has a few snake stories. I didn't encounter as many serpents in Tanganyika as I did as a boy growing up in the Ozarks, but more drama, fear, and excitement resulted. Most African snakes were poisonous, whereas most of the hillbilly snakes which populated my childhood were harmless.

Hooded black cobras thrived in Irambaland and weren't shy about coexisting with humans. They produce a venom which kills in a few minutes. Some cobras also have the nasty habit of spitting their venom several feet with a fair degree of accuracy. Although not lethal, cobra venom in the eyes has much the same effect as a close encounter with tear gas. I once treated a young woman who had been sprayed in the face by a large cobra. She was brought to us holding her eyes, crying, and writhing in pain. Only after washing her eyes, instilling anesthetic eye drops and injecting morphine did her anguish subside. Her eyes were red for twenty-four hours but she had no long-term damage.

Eggs are a part of the cobra's diet. A missionary wife was disturbed by a commotion in their chicken-house. She was horrified to discover a huge black cobra swallowing the last of several eggs. The number consumed could easily be determined by counting the egg-shaped bulges on the snake's upper body. Our friend didn't stay around long enough to count them. She rushed off to get her husband. By the time they returned, the invader had disappeared, eggs and all.

One morning our family was eating breakfast on our screened-in porch at Iambi. Suddenly one of the children shouted, "Snake! Snake!" The lower three feet of the porch was constructed of rough field stones mortared together with cement. A small snake lay coiled comfortably in a recess in this wall, waiting hopefully for breakfast. Our Iramba servant, Danielsoni, identified our visitor as a baby cobra. Fearless Elly rushed over before we could stop her and put her nose just inches away from the snake's head. She wanted to get a better look! Danielsoni rushed to the kitchen for a broom. Afraid to face the snake because he said it would spit in his eyes, he cautiously stepped up to creep along the ledge. When he was directly over the invader, he killed it with the broom handle.

Most of the man/serpent encounters in our corner of the tropics involved puff adders. These slow-moving nocturnal pit vipers resemble sawed-off inflated rattlesnakes without the rattles. They make their living by waiting patiently along the trails of mice and rats. Unsuspecting humans, blundering along in the dark, step on them with inevitable consequences. I treated over a dozen puff adder bites, all on the lower leg. The venom destroys the tissue surrounding the bite, resulting in ugly wounds which take weeks to heal and leave ghastly scars.

One night a healthy young man was bitten just above the ankle. All of his toes except the big one became gangrenous and had to be amputated. Weeks later, after the wounds had healed, he asked me to remove the big toe because it was terribly painful to walk with all of his weight impacting that side of his foot. Instead, we managed to make him a sandal from a rubber tire which put most of the weight on the ball of the foot with less strain on the remaining toe.

As far as we knew, no puff adder bites in our area were fatal. At night we walked carefully always carrying a flash light or lantern. One evening a friend drove up to our front door to pick up a bicycle. He shouted, "Don't come out the door! There's a big puff adder lying on your front steps! I'll return in the morning for the bike." Our serpent visitor was gone in the morning.

The African python stands alone in the snake world because of its gargantuan proportions. They grow up to thirty feet in length and weigh over one hundred pounds. They weren't as prevalent in our open savanna country as in the rain forest, but did inhabit the rock formations surrounding Kiomboi and Iambi.

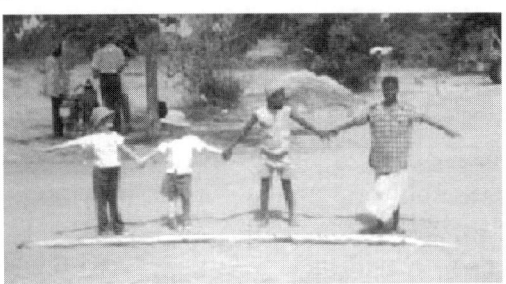

A young man was tending his small flock of goats in the vicinity of a dry riverbed near our home. One afternoon he noticed that a kid was missing. He discovered signs of a telltale struggle in the sand. He followed the trail until it disappeared into a crevice formed by the boulders along the waterway. He waited there with his bow and arrow from dawn to sunset for two days. On the third day, when the python emerged, he killed it with an arrow through the neck. It was only thirteen feet long but weighed at least eighty pounds. He brought it to our house for exhibition. Elly and Dan were duly impressed and had their picture taken with the biggest snake they had ever seen.

Some of the older spectators of this show indicated disapproval that one of their young men had taken the life of a python. In the animistic religion of some tribes the ancestral spirits inhabiting snakes were thought to be threatening to humans. They believed that killing the snake was likely to bring disastrous consequences.

When Adeline and I visited the Nairobi zoo in 1987, we saw a newly captured twenty-five-foot python which the game department had just brought to the reptile garden. A week later on the front page of one of the daily newspapers, an article reported that the people in the valley in which the snake had been caught were up in arms. For years they had paid homage to this serpent. Now her spirit would certainly be angry and bring great trouble upon them if this venerable reptile was not returned to her home.

African mambas, the most dreaded snakes in our region, grow up to fourteen feet in length. Several sub-species range in color from green to brown to black. They are adept at catching birds and glide swiftly through the forest sometimes leaping from tree to tree. Their deadly venom rapidly kills animals as large as cattle.

The only snakebite fatality of which we were aware during our time in Tanganyika was inflicted by a mamba. At one of our mission stations a boy chased a rabbit into a hole. He inserted his arm into the opening and immediately withdrew it with a five-foot mamba attached to his hand. The snake coiled around his arm and continued chewing on the hand. Friends rescued him and rushed him to the nearby missionary's home. Already the lad was having respiratory difficulty. After a tourniquet had been applied, he was loaded into the Jeep to rush him to the hospital. Just as they drove away, he stopped breathing. Resuscitation was unsuccessful. Death came less than fifteen minutes after the fateful encounter.

At Iambi we lived through our own mamba adventure. For several days we had noticed that the Africans were avoiding a path from our house to the hospital which passed a large rock formation. One morning Margaret walked by the rocks. She ran quickly to the house and tearfully told us that a snake had struck out at her, barely missing her leg. I grabbed a heavy hoe and hurried out. Elly was already running ahead of me. Our friend, Pastor Simeon Petro, caught her and pulled her away from the rocks. We put her in the house and ordered her not to come out until given permission. She was furious!

Hurrying back to the rocks I spotted a brown tail and grabbed it. Using considerable force, I was able to pull out a four-foot length of reptile and decapitate it. At that moment another snake emerged and headed straight for me. I was fortunate in being able to get him before he got me. My victims were identified as mambas, probably a courting pair.

Elly, released from house arrest, was angry at missing out on the action. The funeral of her little friend Martin Luther Gunda was held later that afternoon. I told her that we would have had two funerals that day if the snake had bitten her. Her immediate response was, "Oh, you wouldn't have had mine today; you would have waited until tomorrow!" In adult life she wouldn't be caught dead near a live snake. Maybe that's why she moved to Alaska where there are none.

We wondered why the Africans hadn't told us about these dangerous snakes near our house. I felt slightly heroic in dispatching them, but nobody outside of my family congratulated me. One of our Iramba medical workers told me that the mamba was still held in awe and reverence by many of his people. They left offerings of milk near mamba habitat at night. If the milk was gone in the morning the spirits of the serpents were appeased. The possibility that other creatures of the night might have consumed the milk wasn't considered. I could see that I still had much to learn but felt no remorse about destroying the nasty creatures who had endangered Margaret.

28. AARDVARKS AND TERMITE TOWERS

Picturesque anthills dotting the landscape stand out as prominent features of an East African panorama. They appear much like miniature volcanoes up to twenty feet in height and assume the color of the soil from which they are constructed. Ventilation shafts several inches in diameter extend from the central peaks down to the underground living quarters. On cold mornings I have seen wisps of condensed moisture erupting out of these chimneys, making the volcano analogy even more apt. To reach inaccessible food, termites construct clay tubes above ground through which the workers can pass without being exposed to their enemies.

Each anthill represents the fortress domain of a single king and queen termite with hundreds of thousands of their subjects who are also their sons and daughters. The royal father does not die after mating but lives on as a founder and co-ruler of the kingdom. Termites are often called white ants but they are actually more closely related to grasshoppers and cockroaches. They play an important role in tropical ecology with their ability to consume and digest the cellulose in dead wood, grass, and leaves. They fill an ecological niche similar to the soil building earthworms of the temperate climates.

Termites love paper and will devour an unattended book in a short time. One might say that they are fast readers with complete digestion of the printed word!

Only a few tropical woods such as ebony and mahogany are termite-resistant. Using any other lumber for construction is folly. At Kiomboi we built a sign from pine boards out of a packing crate which we mounted on the road near the hospital. One of our African workers predicted that our work of art would soon disappear.

Within a few weeks, termites had completely consumed it leaving only a few shreds of wood scattered on the ground.

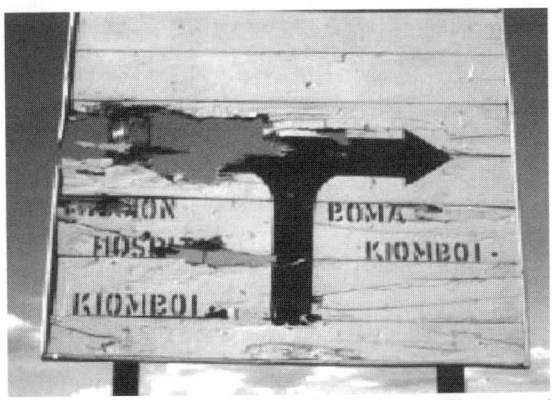

Near our house at Iambi, a single-lane dirt road passed through a cleft between two huge rock formations. A colony of termites began building their castle on the edge of the road at its narrowest point. Soon their construction began encroaching on the roadway, making it difficult to pass through with a car. Before long it would have effectively blockaded four-wheeled vehicle traffic. Something had to be done.

Our African friends informed us that the only sure solution was to destroy the queen. With picks and shovels we began digging toward the royal headquarters underground. The clay walls of the termite city were like concrete. We sweated profusely as we picked away at the protective walls which had been laboriously fabricated by countless tiny workers mixing their saliva with the red volcanic soil. Every time we broke into a passageway, thousands of the soldier termites rushed out to protect their domain. They did not aggressively attack their human invaders but inflicted nasty bites if they reached any part of one's anatomy. I wished that we had had some dynamite or power equipment. The excavation, which lasted two days, created an impressive crater four-feet deep. Finally, one of the workers named Amosi shouted triumphantly as his pick broke into the brood chamber. In a few moments he reached down and lifted out the queen mother.

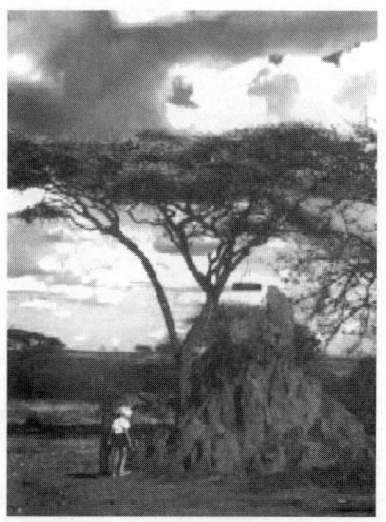

I was astounded to see a grotesque, sausage-shaped white blob as large as my index finger. Amosi handed it to me for closer inspection. I experienced a sense of reverence and awe. Here in my hand I held the germinal source of all of that life and activity. The creative forces of this small mass of protein produced thousands of new lives every day. She contained all the genetic wisdom to construct and maintain a massive purposeful colony, housed for years in a magnificent fortress. Her offspring also provided rich nourishment to countless other creatures, large and small. Amosi brought me out of my reverie as he reclaimed his prize. He would take it home, roast it over the fire and have it as a tasty appetizer before supper. Somehow I felt like the participant in a mass murder of major proportions. As predicted, the colony withered away and our road hazard was permanently removed.

Humans are not the only creatures involved in tropical termite control. Some species depend on termites as a principal source of their livelihood. In my early boyhood I read about one such termite terminator, the aardvark, or earth pig. It was so named by the early Dutch immigrants to South Africa because of its appearance and life style. As a boy, I thought that it must be important because aardvark appeared as the very first word and picture in the dictionary. I even had a recurring fantasy which featured a friendly aardvark and wondered if I would ever get to see one.

A few decades later, my fantasies came to life through an accident which was both dramatic and sad. As I was driving home one night, an animal dashed across the road in front of me. I was cruising along at about 40 MPH and couldn't avoid a jolting collision which produced a sickening thud. The resulting impact threw my head against the windshield dazing me for just a moment. When I stepped out of the Volkswagen van, the headlight beams revealed my very first, and very dead aardvark. It looked exactly like the picture in the dictionary.

It was huge, weighing about a hundred pounds. I examined the formidable claws and powerful shoulder muscles with which it burrows into termite colonies and could understand why aardvarks are reputed to be the best diggers in the animal world. Most astounding to me was my victim's pink sticky tongue, pencil-thin, but projecting more than a foot ahead of the snout. When it breaks through the tough walls of a termite nest, the aardvark uses this marvelous prehensile instrument to harvest all the insects in reach. Rarely do they destroy the colony completely and the termites are able to make repairs in short order.

I considered bringing the forlorn carcass home, but didn't think Adeline would take kindly to the idea of adding roadkill aardvark to the family menu. Actually the meat is highly prized, allegedly tasting much like good lean pork.

Aardvarks aren't alone in depending heavily on termites for their diets. Aardwolfs are closely related to hyenas but are much smaller with tiny teeth and weak jaws best suited for eating insects. They are strictly nocturnal, hunting during the hours of the termite workers' most active foraging expeditions. Chimpanzees have developed the tool-making skill of stripping the leaves from a narrow twig, poking it into the termite hill, and licking off the little creatures which have attacked the stick. Hedgehogs also love ants and termites, as do birds and other vertebrate species. Several types of predatory insects harvest termites as an important part of their diet.

Once each year a termite colony produces a large crop of winged reproductive males and females. These do not compete with the reigning king and queen but fly forth to establish new colonies. On a specific day, the young princes and princesses all crawl up the central shaft of the anthill and take off in such numbers that it appears that a cloud of smoke is issuing from the little volcanoes. Our Iramba friends considered flying termites a special delicacy to supplement the protein in their diets. When the mounds spewed forth their living smoke, there was great excitement as old and young alike rushed around trying to catch as many as possible. Some of our sickest patients abandoned their hospital beds and rushed out to join the gold rush.

One of our doctors had spent two hours skin-grafting burns which covered much of a young man's body. The patient was bandaged carefully and ordered to stay quiet for several days. That very afternoon the termites flew, and the young fellow rushed out to capture his share of the goodies. In a few moments of violent activity, all of the bandages were loosened and the skin grafts completely destroyed.

After collection, the termites were cooked and eaten with great relish. We did not discourage this practice because our African friends needed every bit of protein available. One method of preparation was to impale the insects on a grass stem in the form of a miniature shish kebab. This was then roasted over the fire. On a productive ant day one of my favorite elderly patients was preparing this gourmet delight over a tiny fire near the hospital. He insisted that I sample his wares. Of course I couldn't offend him, so with a little hesitation, accepted his offer. To my pleasant surprise, the crunchy little morsels tasted much like fried shrimp with a bit of a walnut flavor.

Abandoned African anthills still serve many purposes. Other animals, birds, and insects use them for homes and observation platforms. They also form identifiable landmarks in an otherwise featureless plain. Several times I was able to use them as concealment while hunting. Before the tropical sun is directly overhead at mid-day, and again later in the afternoon, animals rest in the cooling shade cast by termite mounds. At noon these shadows all but disappear.

All things considered, African termites are marvelous and fascinating creatures. I will always remember the day I held that termite queen in my hand. Her ancestors have had a major impact on this planet for millions of years and their countless progeny will continue to do so as long as Mother Earth continues to meet their needs.

29. FEATHERED FRIENDS

When I reminisce about days in Africa, I invariably see and hear birds of all sizes, shapes and colors. I was enthralled by the morning symphony of bird songs emanating from the trees and hills around me. I could identify only a few of them. Not being a scientific bird watcher, I simply enjoyed their music and was fascinated by their lifestyles.

TV soundtracks often include the songs of different avian species. The most frequently heard African bird music is that of several species of doves. Their plaintive soothing calls evoked nostalgic memories of the mourning doves of my Ozark childhood. Another favorite of the filmmakers is the call of the rain bird whose pealing three-note song clearly announces, "It-will-rain! It-will-rain!" These secretive creatures are difficult to spot, concealing themselves skillfully in the trees. Many times I tried to visually locate them but was never successful. The raucous, repetitive cacaphony of the hornbill species, rising to a harsh crescendo, is also frequently featured on video soundtracks.

The bee-bird was one of the favorites of our Iramba friends for obvious reasons. One day while I was out hunting, one of my African companions asked me to stop the jeep. He jumped out and followed a small bird flitting from tree to tree, always in the same direction. We hurried after him for perhaps a half-mile. Finally the bird perched in a branch above us and chattered as if trying to tell us something. Our human guide spotted a nearby hollow tree around which many bees were flying. He soon started a fire by twirling the point of a hardwood fire stick into a dry piece of wood. Green twigs and leaves were added to produce thick smoke. He picked up the burning branches and directed the smoke toward the hole in the tree, sedating the bees. With his machete, he enlarged the hole, reached in his bare hand, and began pulling out honeycombs. Although stung several times, he seemed oblivious to the pain. One chunk of honeycomb filled with bee larvae was left near the tree in which the bee bird was perched. This served as a generous reward for leading us to our tasty treat. As we walked away, I looked back and saw our benefactor fly down to enjoy his well-earned feast.

Brightly colored birds abound in East Africa. Many consider the lilac-breasted roller to be the most beautiful of all. The iridescent pinkish-violet breast is set off by the elegant shades of blue on the rest of the body. The name derives from the startling flight of the male rollers. In their courtship display, they perform exciting aerial acrobatics with tumbles and rolls which seem to excite the females of the species. I once had the opportunity to witness a handsome specimen performing brilliantly for his lady-love.

Another entertaining show which we enjoyed on several occasions was the spectacle of hundreds of multicolored parakeets flying in to a water hole. They chattered noisily in a waterside tree before they cautiously flew down to have their daily drink. We watched African boys capture them by coating the small branches of trees with a special sticky sap. When the birds perched on these twigs from which they couldn't extricate their feet, they were captured unharmed to be sold. They would spend the rest of their lives in captivity.

The starling species in Africa put their plain black American cousins to shame with their colorful attire. One of our missionary friends was conducting a brief morning devotional service for a dozen African workers. During the message, a handsome orange-breasted yellow-eyed starling alighted on a rock not twenty feet from me. I had never seen the likes of this beautiful creature before and was mesmerized. When Pastor Bob finished and said, "Let us pray!" all folded their hands and shut their eyes; that is, everybody but me. I clasped my hands together but couldn't keep my eyes off that elegant bird. I was seated next to an intelligent but deaf-mute sixteen-year-old lad who was called Bubu. Bubu is the Swahili word for one who can neither hear nor speak. His ability to communicate was limited because he had had no formal sign language training, but he was incredibly quick at learning by demonstration or example. During the prayer time, he noticed that I had neither closed my eyes nor bowed my head, so he gave me a sharp elbow to the ribs. He was obviously shocked that I was acting like a heathen. Of course, I then assumed a reverent posture. Bubu taught me a lesson, but I still find elegant birds mighty distracting.

Not all African birds are beautiful. One of my favorites, the marabou stork, is also probably the most homely. Adeline teases me about my affinity to these ugly creatures, but I respond by saying, "Where would we pediatricians be if we didn't have storks to provide us with babies?" Whenever the opportunity arose, I invariably took more pictures of marabous than any other wildlife. This ungainly creature with its oversized bill, cold staring eyes, and nearly bald head is usually considered an uncouth scavenger who gathers with the vultures at scenes of death. Observers have indicated, however, that much of his diet is obtained by patient hunting of lizards, snakes and small mammals.

Vultures are in some ways even more repellent than marabou storks. They are, in fact, marvelous creatures who fill an important niche in the ecosystem. Some have developed unique skills to help them make a living. Egyptian vultures are often classified as one of the few sub-human species who have learned to use tools. They are unable to open ostrich eggs with their bills, but somewhere along the line developed a strategy which almost suggests true intelligence. They select tennis-ball sized rocks and pound the ostrich eggs until they break. Some are said to fly into the air with their rocks and drop them onto the eggs.

Vultures are gifted with incredible visual acuity and can spot a potential meal from miles away. One day I was hunting with American friends visiting Africa. We shot a male impala which we were preparing to retrieve when our African guide spotted a herd of hartebeest at least a mile away across the open savanna. As far as we could see, not another creature was in sight. One of the hunters was anxious to collect a set of hartebeest horns, so we drove close enough to stalk and bag one. In less than thirty minutes we returned to retrieve the impala. As we drew near, we were shocked to see at least twenty huge vultures huddled around the carcass, completing their meal. All that remained was skin and skeleton. From where had they come, and how did so many of them arrive so quickly? One of them was probably watching us crazy human hunters from high above and was delighted to see us abandon our kill. As he honed in on this feast, his buddies from miles around could see that he was swooping down and joined him in short order.

On one occasion we had the opportunity to watch a pair of white and black hornbills courting in a sausage tree. Soon they proceeded to build their home in the hollow fork of that same tree. When they were finished, we observed the male sealing his mate into the nest with a wall of mud, leaving only a small hole through which he could feed her. We were fascinated to watch him skillfully perform this construction project with his ungainly banana-shaped bill, delicately smoothing out the opening to just the right size. This afforded effective protection against predators. Even if a snake tried to enter, the nesting mother could block the entryway with her large bill from the inside. We weren't there to see the outcome, but our friends watched Papa hornbill feed his mate through the hole and break down the mud barrier and release the mother when the babies had hatched. Both adults were kept busy in relays, feeding their hungry offspring until the two fledglings emerged and flew off with their parents. Their human neighbors weren't happy that the green tomatoes from the nearby garden became one of the favorite dishes on the hornbill menu.

Ostriches always fascinated us in the wild. Their numbers are decreasing because of human encroachment upon their habitat, but several factors have prevented their becoming an endangered species. This largest of all living birds has a life span of up to eighty years. They are considered stupid, and indeed their brains are no larger than their eyeballs, but certain instincts and their lifestyle favor survival. Since they can live for days without water, many of them occupy deserts which are unfit for most other creatures. Their twenty-five-foot strides enable them to outrun most predators at speeds of up to fifty miles an hour. For defense they have a vicious kick which has been known to break the leg of a horse. Safety also lies in numbers. A dominant male attracts a cluster of up to seven hens. Unattached males also tend to gather in groups.

Early one morning while I was out hunting with African companions, we came upon three male eland browsing in the distance. We stalked them carefully until close enough for a good shot from behind a clump of thorn trees. I fired carefully and knocked down one of the three. We were startled to see a handsome male ostrich jump up and run away from a spot behind the trees not thirty feet in front of us. As we moved forward, we discovered the only ostrich nest I saw in

Africa. A scooped out hollow in the ground held at least thirty eggs. We were tempted to take home a couple of the eggs but this practice was forbidden by the game department.

Later we were given an ostrich egg found on our leprosarium grounds which measured six and five inches in its longitudinal and transverse diameters. Those who know say that a single egg makes a generous serving of omelet or scrambled eggs for ten people. The shell is so thick and durable that small predators are unable to break them.

While traveling through the bush, a missionary friend, Hal Faust, found a recently hatched ostrich chick which had become separated from its family. The parents weren't anywhere in sight so the baby was carried home and put in a pen with their chickens. The rescued orphan attached himself to a bantam hen with her own brood of young. She adopted him although he was already twice her size. When we visited Hal and Louise three weeks later, we were treated to the comical parade of the little mother leading her brood of tiny chicks in single file. At the end of the line came the two-foot-tall adopted brother striding along, seemingly careful not to step on his wee siblings. Shortly thereafter he didn't come home after a day of foraging with his adopted family. Ostriches had been seen nearby so it was hoped that he had found his real mother.

These are just a few of my African feathered friends. For the rest of my life I will remember them with a special sense of wonder and awe.

30. CAMPING WITH THE HIPPOS

Adeline and I both came from rural environments but we hadn't done much outdoor camping. In order to fully experience the excitement, drama, and beauty of the great African out-of-doors, it would be necessary to spend some nights in the pori (uninhabited countryside). We soon discovered that the logistics of camping in the tropical bush country were considerably more complicated than one would surmise from watching Gregory Peck and Ava Gardner on one of their idyllic safaris in the movies. For one thing, they didn't have four children under ten years of age. But we persevered, and many of our happiest and most spectacular memories were generated on family camping trips.

Before going on an extended tent safari, we decided it would be wise to have a trial run not too far from our Iambi home. We borrowed a mosquito-proof tent just large enough for our family of six and practiced setting it up in our yard. Since Adeline and I were the only ones who had sleeping bags, she created one for the older children from an old quilt and blanket. We borrowed a screened-in folding safari crib for seven-month-old Martha. We planned menus and packed the necessary food, dishes, and kitchenware in sturdy boxes. Our list also included large containers of boiled water. We brought two single-burner kerosene stoves but expected to do much of the cooking over an open campfire. One thing we didn't have to worry about was rain gear. After the monsoon rains were over, we could count on dry weather for several months.

Everything was arranged in the back of our enclosed one-ton Jeep truck. I made certain that we had a spare tire plus a sturdy jack, air pump, and tire-patching material. Finally, I included two extra five-gallon cans of petrol, otherwise known as gasoline. We were ready to embark on our first trial camp-out.

Off we went early one sunny afternoon. Our objective was Lake Basuto thirty miles due east of Iambi on a little-used shortcut to the main road to Arusha. I wasn't worried about getting lost because we were heading directly east toward Mt.

Hanang, a conspicuous inactive volcano standing along the Rift Valley. Our progress was slowed by the roughness of the tracks which at some points were barely visible. Nobody seemed to mind the bumpy ride because exotic creatures were almost constantly in view.

Several times we stopped to get a better view of the groups of impala, wildebeest, zebra, gazelle and giraffe. On one occasion, a family of ostriches raced across the road in front of us. Guinea fowl and grouse-like francolin startled us as they flew up in front of the car. Our trip, which appeared so short on the map, took nearly three hours, but finally we saw the glint of sunlight on water in the distance.

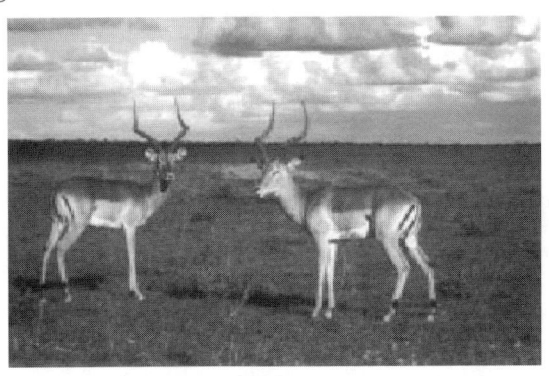

Savannah Royalty

Lake Basuto, one-half mile in diameter, is ringed with picturesque flat-topped acacia trees. Being the only permanent body of standing water for miles around, it is a focal point for a wide variety of creatures. We selected a campsite fifty yards from the water in the shade of a large tree. While we were setting up our tent, a herd of cattle, sheep, and goats was brought to drink by their nomadic Barabaig herdsmen. The group included several small boys who immediately cast aside their garments and began frolicking in the water. Our children were itching to join them, but I vehemently vetoed that proposal because we had heard that this lake was infested with the parasites which cause schistosomiasis. Near the opposite shore we spotted what appeared to be a cluster of gray rocks until we noted that some of them were moving. Dan wasn't sure whether they were hippomuspotuses or hippopotamuses. I just hoped that they stayed on their side of the lake because they are aggressive and dangerous.

At dusk I lit the pressure lantern and we enjoyed our supper around a crackling campfire. Soon we were all ready to settle into the tent for the night. I zipped up our screens before the nocturnal malaria-transmitting mosquitoes became active. We sang several of the children's favorite songs and they said their bedtime prayers, one of which included a petition to keep us safe from the wild animals. As we tried to settle down, a lion roared in the distance. This was followed by a series of eerie hyena calls which seemed to originate from a family group hunting and foraging around the edge of the lake. The most impressive night music came from the herd of hippos as they came out of the water to graze on the tall grass. They blasted out a rumbling bass chorus which had some of the sonic qualities of an army of bullfrogs amplified a hundred times. I was relieved that the sound was obviously moving farther away on the other side of the lake. Instead of being alarmed at these calls of the wild, the children seemed pleasantly excited and fascinated. Later, Margaret told me that she was a little worried, but didn't want to admit it. Snug and safe in our tent, we all slept well through the night.

We were awakened by the early morning sunlight shining through the screen of the tent. A cool brisk trade wind from the east mandated the warmest clothes we had brought along. During the dry season this steady breeze blows almost constantly from that direction and can be uncomfortably cold, with temperatures in the fifties. We heard waterfowl honking in the water nearby so I sneaked out with my shotgun and brought down a plump Egyptian goose. We would take this treat back to Iambi to enjoy later that week. Adeline cooked a hearty breakfast of scrambled eggs and a special treat of Danish canned bacon. While we were eating, we watched flocks of birds coming to drink and heard the wonderful sounds they made as they greeted the new day. A hundred yards away a mother warthog cautiously led her three half-grown piglets to the water. While they were drinking, she was startled by a noise from our campsite and rushed off with her offspring following closely in single file. They all ran with tails erect like car radio antennae.

After our morning meal and dish washing chores we settled down to enjoy the day. Margaret and Elly got out their dolls and strapped them to their backs with carrying cloths. Instead of playing house they went on safari. Dan did the same thing with his cloth monkey. I settled down with a book but found my attention diverted by a troop of monkeys in the trees near us. They noisily scolded us for invading their territory.

After lunch we all took a relaxing siesta. Later the children resumed their play activities while Adeline and I had a leisurely cup of coffee. As the sun sank lower, we broke camp and began our return to Iambi. A magnificent sunset soon faded into darkness and the tropical night engulfed us while we were still several miles from home. We played the exciting game of trying to identify the animals belonging to the eyes picked up by the headlights of our Jeep. Most often these luminous orbs belonged to nocturnal kangaroo-hares about the size of American jack rabbits. The children were amused to watch them hopping along on their hind legs much like the Australian creatures for which they were named. Farther along, I stopped briefly by the rock formation where I had seen a beautiful adult cheetah when I had driven this road a few nights earlier. On this occasion we weren't so fortunate so we continued homeward. Martha was asleep in Adeline's arms as we finally drove up to our house at Iambi. Our first trial camping safari had been an unqualified success. We were looking forward to more extensive adventures in the African pori.

31. ADVENTURES IN THE SOUTHERN HIGHLANDS

For our first major African vacation in August of 1958, we planned a tour of the beautiful mountainous region of southwest Tanganyika known as the Southern Highlands. We chose this area for several reasons. One incentive was my desire to visit Makete, the well-established leprosy settlement near Mbeya. Last but not least was my eagerness to try out the trout fishing in the Livingston Mountains.

Our first one-night camping trip to Lake Basuto had gone smoothly. We realized, however, that a two-week, one thousand-mile trip over rough roads with four small children would be a bit more challenging. With Adeline's efficient planning and direction, we loaded our Jeep one-ton truck. Included were all the items we had carried on our one-day camp-out, only in larger quantities. Of course, I didn't forget my fishing tackle. Previous unhappy experiences prompted me to include an extra spare tire. In the middle of all these loads we prepared a seat for our big girls, Margaret, nine, and Elly, seven. They wouldn't have seat belts but the bed of the truck was boxed in with screened sides.

We headed south through Singida that first morning, making good time until I noticed that our generator wasn't functioning. We drove back twenty miles to Singida where the East Indian garage mechanic installed a rebuilt alternator. Again we headed south. At dusk we reached Itigi which had a government rest house with rustic accommodations where we spent the first night of our vacation.

In the morning we started out early on the unpaved, rough, corrugated road. Most of the way we passed through thick thorn bush country with occasional clearings occupied by small villages. We traveled south for three hundred miles without finding a single filling station. At a Catholic mission we were able to purchase enough petrol to ensure our reaching Mbeya. From dawn till dusk we met only four other vehicles. We were disappointed in not seeing any wild animals. Undoubtedly they were all around us but concealed by the thick brush.

As we neared Mbeya the countryside became more mountainous and green. We drove through hills covered with coffee trees and tea plantations. It looked as if we would reach our destination by nightfall. Suddenly, without warning, our brakes failed completely. I was terrified! We were heading down an incline and picking up speed rapidly when I spotted a side road heading uphill off to the right. I was barely able to make the turn. We coasted upwards to a stop just like we would have on a runaway truck ramp on the steep descent of an American freeway. Had this road not been there, I'm certain we would have accelerated to uncontrollable speed because the Jeep transmission was difficult for me to double-clutch and slow down. We later discovered that this was the only side road for miles and miles. It seemed miraculous that we happened onto it just when we did.

We found ourselves brakeless, sitting high on the mountainous eastern wall overlooking a branch of the Great Rift Valley. Somehow we had to descend over a thousand feet to the city of Mbeya in the valley ten miles below. The sun was low in the west and darkness was imminent. A brisk and chilly wind was blowing so Margaret and Elly were getting cold in the back of the truck. We decided that all six of us should be together in the cab. Adeline held Martha on her lap and Dan sat on an empty five-gallon kerosene tin in front of her. I was in the right-hand driver's seat with Margaret and Elly snugly packed in the middle.

I breathed a silent prayer as I put the Jeep in the lowest tractor gear to crawl down the tight hairpin curves. No guard rails existed on either side of the road. We proceeded slowly about a mile to the steepest part of the descent. Suddenly, the transmission slipped out of gear and, try as I might, I could not re-engage it. We picked up speed rapidly. I was desperate! There was an embankment to the right so I turned the front wheels sharply into it. The right front wheel climbed up the bank, and our vehicle rolled slowly over onto its left side. Adeline, Martha and Dan were underneath with the rest of us on top. I managed to reach up to open the driver's door, climbed out, lifted up each of the children and finally helped Adeline emerge. None of us suffered as much as a scratch or a bump. We were relieved that we had all been together in front. The children calmly accepted our rollover with absolutely no crying or screaming. The vehicle suffered little damage and our supplies were intact except for a few broken eggs.

If we had gone fifty yards farther, we would have encountered a steep curve to the left which we couldn't possibly have negotiated. We would have certainly ended up on the rocks hundreds of feet below. We could see the rusty remains of a bus and a truck which had long ago missed the curve and gone over the cliff. I commented that, if we hadn't turned over when we did, all of us would have been down there on the rocks. Our one-of-a-kind Elly nonchalantly commented, "Oh well! Then we all would have been up in heaven with God!" There was no doubt in her mind. We could count on her optimism to discern the silver lining of every cloud.

We lit a hurricane lantern and wrapped the children in blankets. I placed two debes (metal kerosene cans) on the curve fifty yards above us as warning signals to descending vehicles. Adeline and I unloaded our tangled mass of supplies and prepared a space for the family to huddle together in the back of the tipped-over truck. By then it was almost totally dark and we shivered in the cold wind. Seeing the fires of a village far below us, I decided to walk down the road to seek help. I hadn't gone more than a quarter of a mile when I heard cars coming down the mountain. My immediate fear was that they might speed around the curve and crash into our vehicle. I ran back up the road, arriving breathlessly just in time to see two Landrovers stopping to give us aid. They had seen my caution signal.

A party of several men from Mbeya had been out hunting buffalo in the mountains. Among them were the European owner of the only garage in town and a Sikh police officer. The former assured us that he could rescue our truck in the morning, and the latter, that I should come in to his office to file a report. They told us that they were probably the last vehicles coming over that road until morning. They packed all of us and part of our luggage into the two Landrovers and drove us down to the Mbeya hotel where we settled in comfortably for the next three days.

In the morning the garageman took me with him to retrieve our vehicle and tow it into town. The policeman took care of the accident report without giving me a bad time.

Mbeya was an important administrative and trade center with a population of five thousand which included five hundred Europeans. We enjoyed the opportunities for a little sightseeing and shopping while our truck was being repaired.

On the fourth morning we loaded our Jeep and drove thirty miles through thick fog to Makete Leprosarium. I spent two days checking out the treatment program which I described in the chapter on leprosy. Adeline caught up on household chores at the guest house while the children enjoyed playing with the family of the British doctor-in-charge.

From Makete we drove through gorgeous green mountain terrain to camp one night on the beach at the northern tip of Lake Nyasa, now known as Malawi. This large body of water lies in the southern extension of the Great Rift Valley and is famous for having many species of cichlid fish which are prized by tropical fish devotees throughout the world. Just before we reached Lake Nyasa, we took a short side trip to one of the most beautiful landscapes I have ever witnessed, a perfectly circular clear blue crater lake nestled in tropical greenery.

On the way back north we stopped for two nights at a rustic fishing camp which I had reserved from the Mbeya Trout Association. The Kiwira River had been stocked with rainbow trout fingerlings hatched from fertile eggs imported from Europe years earlier. We found adequate sleeping space for the six of us in a grass-thatched rondeval. A nearby kitchen even came with a combination cook and handy man.

We arrived at dusk too late to fish, but I was able to scout the stream a bit in the fading light. I had fished in the Ozarks, the Bavarian Alps, the Rocky Mountains and the brooks of Northern Minnesota, but this was the most exotic setting of all. At dawn the next morning, I was out wading the crystal clear stream, enchanted by the music of the rushing water and tropical bird songs. A fish attacked my dry fly on the second cast and I set the hook so hard I broke my leader. On the next try I was more careful and had the thrill of landing a beautiful fat rainbow trout. Over the next hour I caught three more, all 12-15 inches in length, plump, and brilliantly colored.

I hurried home to show off my catch. After breakfast, I snapped a picture of Martha admiring my trophies. As I was getting ready to clean the fish, the African cook relieved me of the creel. He not only cleaned them but also fried them to perfection for lunch and supper. I fished for several more hours and caught additional trout which I released because we already had all we could eat.

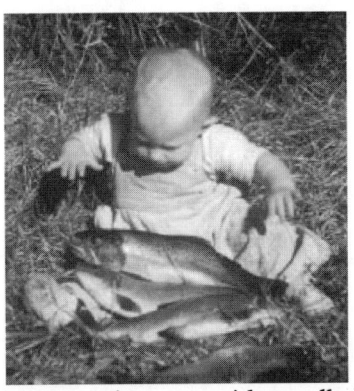

On the following morning we said goodbye to the fishing camp and headed north. The Jeep's alternator malfunctioned again so we stopped at the garage in Mbeya. Our mechanic friend who had rescued us on the escarpment determined that we needed a new voltage regulator which he would be able to install the following day. We checked into the hotel once more. We had just settled into our room when a barefoot African porter dressed in a flowing white gown and bright red fez appeared at our door. He reported that guests, who had just checked in, had seen our name on the hotel register and asked to see us. We were surprised because we didn't know anybody in Mbeya and none of our missionary colleagues had plans to be in Southwest Tanganyika.

We hurried to the lobby, where an elderly American couple greeted us warmly. Eleven years earlier while participating in a medical ROTC training program, I had spent a pleasant weekend with Doc and Mildred Meisch in their home in San Antonio, Texas. They were good friends of one of my favorite aunts. Doc was a retired army colonel and a dedicated big game hunter. He had engaged a white hunter to take him into fabled game territory in the Ruaha valley east of Mbeya.

There he would try to shoot trophy sable antelope, kudu, and oryx to mount on his walls at home.

We had corresponded for a couple of years, then lost track of each other. My aunt had told them that we were in Africa but they didn't even know which country. What a coincidence to cross paths eight thousand miles from home! And it wouldn't have happened if our alternator hadn't gone bad again. We had a great time visiting and sharing meals together. The children enjoyed having grandparent substitutes with whom to interact. Adeline and Mildred went Christmas shopping. It was only August but this would be the last time we would be around any kind of shopping center for the rest of the year.

We were behind schedule for our return trip and didn't get started from Mbeya until late on Saturday afternoon. At Chunya, forty miles north, we stopped to greet friends from Kiomboi, a Scottish miner and his Italian wife, Don and Mimi Mustard. Mimi was the daughter of the Bicchieris, good friends of our mission family, who operated the gold mine near Kiomboi. The Mustards persuaded us to spend the night with them before we embarked on that long lonely road northward. Knowing that Mimi was a wonderful cook made the decision easier. We enjoyed their warm hospitality.

At 7:30 the next morning we started out over the road which alternated between washboard corrugation and foot-deep sand. We didn't take a proper rest stop for five hours because each time we slowed down, tsetse flies swarmed around the cab. Though we didn't see any wild animals, we knew they were there because the tsetse flies wouldn't have been able to complete their life cycle without fresh mammalian blood.

Suddenly we hit a large bump and heard a terrible grinding noise under the hood. An engine mount had broken which caused the fan blades to hit the radiator. We were immediately attacked by hungry tsetse flies so we slowly drove on to a fly-free open area. I jacked up the engine from below and suspended it from the frame with a tow rope. This enabled us to continue, but I didn't dare drive more than 30 MPH. My makeshift repair held up for the rest of the trip. I drove on to the point of exhaustion near midnight. We had been on the road sixteen hours with only short stops for lunch, supper and repairs. We parked at the side of the road, took out all of our loads, spread our sleeping bags on the truck bed, and rested until morning light.

A new day dawned, August 25th, Adeline's birthday. Following a roadside breakfast we gave her a set of flashy earrings which the children and I had bought in Mbeya.

After another hour's drive we arrived at Melanders' mission station south of Singida. Uncle Lud and Aunt Esther were special favorites of our family. They were nearing retirement after spending most of their adult lives in Africa. He had bounced me on his knee when I was a toddler in Northern Tanganyika in 1925. Esther had been a passenger on the Egyptian ship the Zam Zam with my father when it was sunk by the Germans in 1941. The Melanders were famous for making beautiful music together, he on the violin with her piano or accordion accompaniment. They welcomed us warmly into their home.

We were filthy, dressed in the same clothes we had worn since leaving Chunya, but Adeline was wearing her exotic new earrings. We accepted the invitation to use the bathroom to wash and change clothes. They had no running water, but the large bucket contained cloudy, murky liquid from their water hole. A handwritten sign said, "Please pardon our muddy water! The elephants got to the water hole before we did!" Still we felt cleaner and more comfortable after we had washed and put on fresh clothes.

After a cup of Aunt Esther's Swedish coffee and goodies, we embarked on the last leg of our journey to Kiomboi. We stopped for a picnic lunch, our last meal on the road, and time for more birthday celebration. I brought out a tinned fruitcake and candles which I had bought in Mbeya. It was necessary to light the candles in the cab of the truck because the wind was blowing so hard. After we sang "Happy Birthday," Adeline insisted that this had been one of the best birthday celebrations ever. Two more hours of driving brought us safely home.

32. HAVEN OF PEACE

Our second annual vacation found us camping for two weeks on the beach near Dar es Salaam, Tanganyika's capitol city, in August 1959. In Arabic, Dar es Salaam means Place of Peace. The appeal of that fabled metropolis related to the tapestry of its history which had been crafted by powerful African chiefs, Portuguese explorers, Muslim sultans, Arab slave traders, spice merchants, missionaries, German planters and British colonialists.

In 1943 my father, Rev. Ralph Hult, who served as District Mission Superintendent, died and was buried there. In 1958, while attending a mission doctors' meeting in Dar, I retraced the footsteps of the last days of his life. I looked up his friend, Mr. Driver, a British missionary, who had cared for him during his final illness, taken him to the hospital, and later helped make funeral arrangements. I visited the beautiful, palm-shaded Ocean View Hospital, talking to an African male nurse who actually remembered my father's last hours. I was able to locate a retired Indian Muslim bank teller who had become quite fond of his friend, "Bwana Ralph." I attended services at the Lutheran church where he had preached and in which his funeral was conducted. Finally, I located his grave at the attractive European cemetery and spent a quiet hour there, remembering the strong, gentle man whom I had never called by any other name than "Daddy." On our vacation safari, I was looking forward to sharing these experiences with my family.

Preparations for our trip were complicated by Adeline's health. Fourteen days before we were supposed to leave, she miscarried an early pregnancy. After surgery under spinal anesthesia she developed a severe post-spinal headache and was confined to bed for the next ten days. During the two days just before departure, she struggled with the logistics of packing for a three-week camping trip. She was assisted by our two lovely helpers, Wansegamela and Wampumbula. The children were helpful, too. I was kept busy at Kiomboi Hospital right up to the day we left.

We had reserved the more comfortable of the two vehicles at Kiomboi, a Jeep station wagon. By the time we had loaded the supplies for three weeks, it appeared that we might have to leave some of our passengers at home, but Adeline found a spot for everything and everybody.

We had agreed to share this vacation trip with Roly Renner, his wife Marge, and their four sons. We were to meet them in Singida fifty miles from Kiomboi at ten o'clock in the morning. With an early start we managed to make that appointed time. Six hours later the Renners finally arrived, having had car trouble on the way. Their one-ton Jeep truck was completely filled with their supplies, which even included a wood-burning stove.

We had budgeted three days for our five hundred-mile trip to the coast because of the rough dusty corrugated roads. Already delayed, we decided to drive at least the first sixty miles and sleep at the government rest house at Manyoni. Not having to pitch our tents that first night would give us a better start the next morning. Government rest houses provided rustic sleeping accommodations and limited kitchen facilities. We arrived at our destination well after dark, ate a quick meal, and settled in for the night.

On day two, after Marge and Adeline had fed us a breakfast of hot cereal, we embarked soon after sunrise. We had driven only five miles when the Renners' vehicle suffered a flat tire. Roly discovered the culprit to be a large acacia thorn. Within ten minutes after mounting his only spare, another tire went down. This time he had to patch the inner-tube. Soon after we set off again, another tire deflated, again punctured by a thorn. And so it went, with twelve flat tires on the Renner Jeep in the first hundred miles. The day before, they had inadvertently driven under a dead tree with numerous thorns on the ground. These were now working their way through the thin-walled tires. Finally we arrived at Dodoma where Roly was able to buy two replacement tires. No more flat tires slowed our progress.

The road to Dar es Salaam paralleled the trans-Tanganyika railroad. Our children were fascinated to see trains powered by steam locomotives chugging along next to us. The full-throated blasts and wails of their whistles transported me back to childhood days in the Ozarks. We passed through towns with such fascinating names as Kikombo, Mpwapwa, Kimamba, and Bunduki.

We did not find a suitable campsite in the rough terrain of unfamiliar territory so kept on driving until after midnight. Forward progress was suddenly halted when our left front wheel fell off and rolled down the road ahead of us. None of us was injured but we had no choice but to stop for the night. We pitched our tents in the tall grass along the side of the road and bundled up in our sleeping bags for the night. When morning arrived we found ourselves in a desolate landscape of scrubby thorn trees. We were happy to discover that there was no significant damage to our vehicle and were able to find enough spare bolts to remount the wheel.

On our third day we hurried on, climbing into picturesque mountain terrain. We descended onto the coastal plain soon after we passed through the large town of Morogoro.

We arrived in Dar es Salaam just in time to catch the last ferry across the harbor to get to our campsite on the beach five miles southeast of the city. We were fascinated to enter an environment of abundant moisture after two years in relatively waterless Irambaland. The white sandy beach, washed by incoming waves from the deep blue Indian Ocean, was framed by stately palm and delicately needled evergreen trees. We had driven into a veritable paradise. We pitched our tent under a spreading casuarina tree fifty yards from the water's edge and ate our supper around a glowing campfire. Bedtime came early that night. The rhythmic music of the surf breaking on the nearby beach soon lulled us to sleep.

In the morning we were pleased to discover that we had this section of the beach completely to ourselves. The nearest human habitation was a fishing village two miles away. The soil was too sandy and infertile for agriculture. We found evidence of a deteriorating mud-brick compound near our tents. Later we were told that this had probably been a holding area for slaves, built by the Arabs a century earlier. A rock-lined well still held fresh clear water. We resisted the temptation of a quick cold drink, using it only after boiling. We dug a US Army style slit trench for our bathroom facility. Adeline and Marge organized an efficient outdoor kitchen which even included an oven in which they baked fresh biscuits.

For the next two weeks we led an idyllic Swiss Family Robinson existence, although we had brought a lot of the better things in life with us. We enjoyed splashing in the balmy waters of the Indian Ocean. With a scuba mask we were able to see some of the bright fish and other colorful underwater creatures. Our children found the sand just perfect for all sorts of construction and excavation. I discovered, to my dismay, that tropical coral is not kind to bare feet.

One day we were enchanted to watch an ancient Arab dhow, with sails billowing in the wind, gliding slowly into Dar es Salaam. Identical vessels had plied these waters for five hundred years. One morning we were entertained by African fishermen making a big sweep with their net through the waters near our camp. They were pleased to sell us a couple of perch-like fish to enrich our menu.

One night after the children had gone to sleep, Adeline and I slipped out of the tent and sat together in the sand just out of reach of the waves. We thrilled at the spectacle of the full tropical moon ascending out of the Indian Ocean. In this exotically romantic setting we renewed our pledge of mutual love.

One morning we drove into the big city to visit my father's grave and tour the sites which had been important in his last days. We stocked up on tangerines, bananas, and mangoes at the colorful African market. By noon we were more than ready to hurry back to our Shangri-La on the beach. We were excited that we had been joined by another missionary family from Irambaland, Les and Ruth Peterson and children. Margaret and Elly hurried to join their friends, Louella and Rachel. Les, who was the acknowledged horseshoe pitching champion of the mission family, had brought his shoes. Roly, Les and I had some lively games much to the amusement of the African villagers as they passed our encampment.

When our vacation days ended, we reluctantly prepared to return up-country. As we packed up our gear, we were horrified to find two scorpions in the corner of the tent under Martha's safari crib. Our return trip to Kiomboi was accomplished safely without a single flat tire. As we look back on our days in Africa, this vacation on the beach is remembered as a special time of happiness, healing, and togetherness for our family.

In 1960 Mother was able to visit Daddy's grave for the first time. When she retired from her missionary service in Bolivia at age sixty-two she made plans to visit us in Africa. She traveled by bus across the Andes to Uruguay, sailed to Capetown, South Africa, on a freighter, and completed the last leg of her journey to Dar es Salaam by plane. We took her to the cemetery and shared special moments as she stood at his last resting place.

Then we took the train to central Tanganyika where she visited with us for four months.

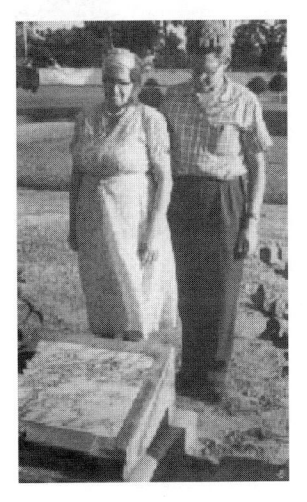

Thirty-seven years later our granddaughter, Heather Ruud, spent the fall term of her junior year at the University of Dar es Salaam. She was busy with her studies as an exchange student but one of her special objectives was to visit her great-grandfather's grave. With the changes in mission staff and African pastors, the location of the burial site had been lost.

Rev. Ralph Kuserow and his wife Carol checked with the grave registration offices but found no record of American missionary deaths in Dar es Salaam. Heather didn't give up her quest. After nearly four months, with the help of African friends, she was successful. She started her letter to us with the words, "I FOUND IT! I FOUND IT!" Then she related the details of the moving moments which culminated in her standing at the graveside of her great-grandfather Ralph.

33. LEARNING TIME IN KAMPALA

In September of 1959 our hospital mail contained an exciting communiqué. UNICEF, a children's division of the World Health Organization, had scheduled a six-day seminar entitled Problems of Child Health and Welfare in East Africa. UNICEF offered to pay part of the expenses of the mission representatives who attended. One of the faculty was to be Dr. D. B. Jelliffe, a leading international authority on tropical pediatrics. He had been Visiting Professor of Pediatrics at Tulane University when I studied tropical medicine there in 1956. He was a stimulating and pragmatic mentor and had taken a special interest in my plans for working in Tanganyika. Dr. Jelliffe had spent most of his professional life working and teaching in Third World countries, including Sudan, Nigeria, India, and Jamaica.

The seminar was to be held at Makerere Medical School, Kampala, Uganda, in late February 1960. I very much wanted to attend. When I informed my colleagues, they suggested that with my pediatric background I was the logical one to go and encouraged me to apply. We eagerly made plans since this would be a great opportunity for Adeline to get away for a much needed rest and change of scenery. Martha would be happy and content to stay with friends at Kiomboi. We anticipated a special time together in a beautiful and fabled region of Africa.

When the hepatitis epidemic swept through our missionary family, Adeline was one of the last victims. After being quite ill, she was just beginning to recover a week before our proposed trip to Uganda. The awareness that she would be in no condition to travel was a crushing blow to her morale. I felt guilty about leaving her, but did go ahead with my plans.

Kampala lies three hundred miles north of Kiomboi. Initially, I thought of the exciting possibility of catching a bus to Mwanza and then taking overnight steamship passage across Lake Victoria. I soon discovered that without more time that route would be unfeasible. Dean Buchanan, our missionary accountant, offered me a ride on a business trip to Nairobi. We made the trip in a VW Beetle in one long day, a safari which usually consumed two days traveling over the atrocious roads. The magnificent views of the Rift Valley, Mount Kilimanjaro and abundant wildlife made the time pass swiftly.

While in the big city, I had an appointment with a British internist, Dr. Winteler, who was concerned that my recovery from hepatitis was slower than it should have been. He suggested that I should take a month's rest before returning to work. That made me feel a little less guilty about leaving my friends short-handed at Kiomboi.

At 9:00 a.m. the next morning, I boarded the East African Railroad passenger train for the twenty-seven hour trip to Kampala. I had read several books and seen movies about the construction of this famous set of tracks. They included accounts of devastating epidemics, man-eating lions, and prodigious engineering feats. I looked forward to experiencing in comfort the results of those painful labors.

As we slowly moved out of Nairobi, the powerful chugging of the steam locomotive, the haunting wail of the whistle, and the rhythmic clackity-clack of the wheels brought back nostalgic memories. We traveled by Lake Nakuru, bordered in pink by a solid mass of flamingos. Wildlife dotted the landscape in all directions. A herd of stately eland in single file trotted alongside the train briefly before disappearing into the forest.

After moving briskly through the countryside, we slowed down almost to a crawl as we climbed up the steep western escarpment of the Rift Valley into the picturesque White Highlands. We passed through well-groomed tea and coffee plantations with hundreds of colorfully clad women hard at work. From horizon to horizon, the earth was painted in varying shades of green, and the sky, a lovely blue. Exotic names identified the towns in which we stopped: Naivasha, Gilgil, Nakuru, Thika, Eldoret.

My seatmate was a young German accountant who had been born in Tanganyika. His parents were among the few German citizens British authorities had permitted to return after being interned in both World Wars. Meals in the dining car were tasty, even with my unhealthy liver. Soon after night fell, I settled into my sleeping berth and was rocked to sleep by the gentle rolling of the train.

When I awoke, we had crossed into Uganda and soon arrived at the bridge crossing the Victoria Nile. A dramatic view of the dam at Owens Falls appeared out of the left windows. This marvel of engineering, completed in 1954 and dedicated by Queen Elizabeth, was projected to raise the water level in Lake Victoria three feet during the next century. Actually, it is a relatively small dam but the British engineers claimed that it would impound 15,000 times more water per square yard of concrete than Boulder Dam on the Colorado River. This hydroelectric project provided virtually all of Uganda's electricity with much left over to export to Kenya and Ruanda-Burundi. As the train rolled over the long-searched-for source of the Nile River, I wondered how many days would pass before some of these molecules of water would complete their long journey northward through Sudan and Egypt finally flowing into the Mediterranean Sea.

From Jinja westward we passed through a heavily populated area. The country-side was intensively cultivated with corn, bananas, plantains, coffee trees, citrus groves, and cotton fields. At that time Uganda was the largest producer of cotton and coffee in the British Empire. Chubby little Ugandans rushed out of their thatched homes to wave and smile as the train rolled by.

Late in the morning, the graceful modern city of Kampala, built on a cluster of seven hills, came into view. Atop three of these elevations were a mosque, a large Anglican church and a Catholic cathedral, symbolic of the religious rivalries which had plagued Uganda's development. We passed many elegant homes as we entered the suburbs. At noon we rolled into the substantial Kampala station, the terminus of the East African Railroad.

A handsome young African in my compartment had become my self-appointed travel guide that morning. He was neatly dressed in a dark suit, white shirt, and tie. Recently graduated from New York University with a degree in economics, he worked for the Cal-Ter Corporation. As we stepped off the train, he offered to transport me to my hotel in his car. I gratefully accepted but became a little uneasy as he whizzed casually through the heavy vehicular, bicycle and pedestrian traffic of downtown Kampala. I shouldn't have worried, for he soon delivered me safely to my destination.

Kampala's Imperial Hotel was the most elegant Victorian edifice I had seen in East Africa. After checking in, I was escorted to my room by a muscular African porter wearing a neat khaki shirt-and-shorts uniform topped off by a bright red fez set at a jaunty angle. My spacious airy room featured a panoramic view of the colorful hotel gardens. Gentle waves of air wafted down from a slowly revolving fan on the high ceiling. I wished that Adeline could have been there to experience this relaxing luxury with me.

I hurried down to the dining room just in time to get in on the hotel's famous ten-course lunch. Space was limited and a friendly Scottish couple invited me to share their table. The gentleman introduced himself as a District Officer from Kenya and his wife as a pediatrician there to attend the seminar. I was delighted; I hadn't had the privilege of conversing with another pediatrician for almost three years. She and I shared with each other the stories of our backgrounds and training in child health. At that time she was working half-time, traveling to a series of clinics for children in her husband's district, plus training Kenyan nurses to conduct well-baby and immunization programs. Our conversation was animated and excited to the extent that I feared that her nonmedical husband might feel excluded. When I apologized to him, he reassured me that he was happy to have his wife find somebody besides himself with whom to share the stories about her little African patients.

After lunch I made a two-hour walking tour of the neighborhoods surrounding the hotel. In 1960 Kampala seemed peaceful and prosperous. Bicycles and motorcycles outnumbered automobiles. Most cars were fairly new and were driven by Africans. Many of the Ugandan male pedestrians were dressed in business suits and walked briskly with their heads held high. On several occasions I was greeted by a cheerful English "Hello!" and a friendly smile.

Most of the African women displayed unique, elaborate hairdos and were dressed in colorful Mother Hubbard dresses. A high percentage of the businesses I passed were owned by East Indians wearing Sikh turbans. (They were later dispossessed and deported by the treacherous Idi Amin regime.) I climbed to the top of the hill on which the modern buildings of Makerere Medical School and Mulago Hospital were situated. Off in the distance, I could see Lake Victoria shimmering in the afternoon sun. As I headed back to the hotel, a crescent moon appeared in the east as the sun neared the western horizon. Walking alone with night descending, I thought of my family three hundred miles to the south in Tanganyika.

Our seminar sessions began on the following morning at Mulago Hospital. The first person I encountered was Dr. Jelliffe who greeted me cordially and recalled our times together in New Orleans four years earlier. He would be serving as chairman and moderator for most of the program over the next five days. The seminar faculty was equally divided between Ugandan and Kenyan physicians and professors from Makerere, and pediatricians and medical officers from the United Kingdom. In 1960, as far as I know, no Tanganyikans had completed medical school. I was anxious to see and hear the indigenous physicians in action and was favorably impressed. Following are a few of the highlights of the seminar.

The British Research Council was conducting an extensive study comparing Bagandan children born and reared in a traditional village with those of the same tribe born to urban, educated, Europeanized parents. Many of the latter group were bottle-fed on a rigid schedule, slept in cribs away from their mothers, were carried about in buggies, and picked up infrequently. Such was the manner in which most American and European babies were reared at the time.

In the tribal setting, the mothers carried the babies on their backs, slept with them, and nursed them at will. Constant maternal presence and attention prevailed. The village babies developed much more rapidly in terms of sitting, standing, walking alone, gaining manual skills, and learning to talk. We watched an amazing movie of an African baby, with a documented age of five months, walking alone at least eight feet across the floor from his grandmother to his mother.

These rural babies maintained this lead over the urban tots for the first two or three years. Thereafter the Europeanized children, with better nutrition, less infection, and more intellectual stimulation, tended to pass them up in most developmental landmarks. Dr. Jelliffe commented that these results suggested the need for a two-way flow of ideas wherein we should adopt the best traditions from both the old and the new patterns of child rearing.

Some of the lectures had moments of high drama, such as the African doctor's account of stopping a terrible polio epidemic in its tracks with the use of the new Sabin oral vaccine. In a report of the effects of obstetrical problems, we heard the astounding story of an African woman, in desperation after hours of agonizing labor, doing a Caesarean section on herself and living to tell about it.

All of us were intrigued by the report of the discovery in Kampala of a previously unrecognized type of childhood cancer by Dr. Burkitt, a brilliant British surgeon. It was the most common form of childhood cancer in Uganda but recognized only sporadically throughout the rest of the world. Today, universally known as Burkitt's lymphoma, it has been the subject of much research leading to a better understanding of the immune system and possible causes of other types of cancer.

Much of the material presented had practical application in dealing with the complex child health problems we faced in Tanganyika. Just a few simple changes in the pattern of nutrition and hygiene could save the health and lives of thousands of African babies, but such steps come slowly and only with persistent repetitive effort.

On the final evening of the seminar, the participants had a group dinner at the Imperial Hotel. I was invited to sit at the table with Dr. Jelliffe and his lovely blonde wife. He gave her much of the credit for his achievements in teaching and research. Also seated at my table were the directors of government medical services in Uganda and New Guinea, the Scottish pediatrician in charge of the big children's hospital in Nairobi, a prominent Arab physician from Zanzibar, and other dignitaries. I wondered what I was doing in such distinguished company.

On the following day, I boarded the train back to Nairobi. As I rode along through the beautiful equatorial landscape, my mind was filled with thoughts about how I could put into practice some of the information presented during the week. I compiled and later duplicated my notes in the hope that they would be of some use to my coworkers in Tanganyika.

As the train rolled through Uganda, I was impressed with this seemingly prosperous and peaceful country and the individual Ugandans I had met. The subsequent tragic chapters in that nation's history have been painful to follow. Much of the progress and accomplishments I witnessed have been destroyed.

After spending a night in a Nairobi guest house, I was eager to get back home. I had a pleasant ride to Arusha with missionary pastor Karl Johanson. Since he had gone to college with my younger brothers and sisters in Nebraska and had been a student pastor in Adeline's home church in Kansas, we had much to talk about.

The last twelve-hour leg of my safari was completed as the only non-African passenger on an ancient and crowded cracker-box bus. Most of the passengers were cheerful and friendly, chattering to each other in a cacophony of languages. I enjoyed visiting in Swahili with a middle school student who declared that he wanted some day to became a "Daktari."

I had brought along a brown bag lunch and was able to purchase unrefrigerated Coca Cola in the villages at which we stopped. No sanitary facilities were available so our journey was occasionally punctuated with pit stops along the road. My tired body was much relieved as we rolled into Singida in a cloud of dust soon after sunset.

What a thrill it was to spot Adeline, holding Martha, waiting for me in the crowd at the bus stop! She had made considerable progress in her recovery from hepatitis. I had experienced an exciting and stimulating week but was both relieved and delighted to be back home in Iramba-Turuland.

34. ARUSHA, MOSHI, AND MACHAME

The clock-tower on the main street of downtown Arusha is allegedly the mid-point on the Capetown-to-Cairo Highway. This picturesque town, nestled at the foot of Mt. Meru, was a special Mecca for our mission family who lived two hundred miles southwest on the Iramba plateau. Arusha provided the nearest shopping center, dentist, and full-service garage, plus a modestly priced hotel. During the dry season the greenery of the mountain topography afforded a welcome relief from our semi-desert landscape.

In August 1960 we embarked on a three-week family vacation safari to Arusha and other sites in beautiful and legendary northeastern Tanganyika. The timing couldn't have been better. I was still recovering from hepatitis, and the hospital schedule had been particularly exhausting. Also, Margaret, Elly, and Dan were on vacation from school. Veda had arranged her vacation schedule so that she could accompany us. We eagerly anticipated those days together in a region which had special significance in our family history thirty years earlier.

The seven of us would be traveling in the relative comfort of the mission-owned Volkswagen van, also known as the Kombi. Unfortunately, this vehicle was mechanically temperamental. I had been requested to see that major work be done on the transmission in Arusha. Our journey began early on the morning of August 25th, Adeline's birthday. We packed up and embarked in high spirits but were barely out of sight of Kiomboi when the engine began sputtering badly and stalled. The gas line to the carburetor was clogged. It took two hours to get it cleared out. Then the transmission began emitting ominous noises if I drove over 40 MPH.

At our first rest stop, Veda and the children eagerly got out a birthday cake which they had smuggled along for an impromptu party for Adeline. The cake was badly misshapen from Adeline's having inadvertently sat on the box as she packed loads into the car. With a quick repair job, the cake didn't appear too disreputable, but lighting the candles in the 30 MPH dry season wind was a real challenge. We formed a human shield around the cake to protect the candles from the wind. After we sang "Happy Birthday," the wind blew out the candles. That was Adeline's second birthday party on the roadside in Africa.

We spent a long dusty day driving north on the unpaved one-lane Capetown to Cairo Highway. We did see much wildlife and admired the profiles of the volcanic peaks, Mt. Hanang and Mt. Meru, as we approached them. To the west we could barely see the eastern rim of Ngorongoro Crater as we drove by beautiful Lake Manyara. The sun had set when we reached our destination, a small furnished guest house at Makumira Seminary outside Arusha. Dean and Elaine Peterson were on hand to welcome us and insisted that we share their evening meal with them.

After breakfast the following morning, Adeline and I were making plans for the day. Our two-and-a-half year old Martha slipped out the door to do some exploring. Thirty minutes later she came crying to the door covered with dust. She had cuts and scratches on her face, hands, and legs. After consoling her, cleaning her up, and dressing her wounds, we asked her to show us what had happened. She led us to the garbage pit behind the house. We were shocked to see a steep-sided ten-foot hole partially filled with garbage, cans, bottles, and broken glass. Martha had apparently approached too close to the edge and fallen in. When we asked how she got out she replied, "Lellow socks!" We tried to get more details but she kept repeating, "Lellow socks!" Then we remembered that the Peterson's cook, a bright friendly young man, had been dressed in shorts and bright yellow socks. We went to the kitchen and asked him. He smiled and acknowledged that he had heard her crying and ran to rescue her. We were amazed that he had been able to negotiate the steep sides and lift her out of the pit on his own. We gratefully expressed our appreciation in Swahili, "Asante sana! Asante sana!" Then I probably scared and embarrassed him when I gave him a quick hug of gratitude. Martha had recently had her tetanus booster so she was well protected. Her injuries healed without infection or scarring.

Later in the day Adeline, who was in the early stages of a pregnancy, began cramping. We drove to the hospital where she miscarried. We were deeply disappointed, more so because she had experienced the same trauma and grief a year before at Kiomboi. We were intensely grateful for Veda's presence and emotional support.

Earlier that day the Petersons and Palms had taken Margaret, Elly, and Dan along with their six children for an exciting visit to Amboseli Game Park. When they hadn't returned by late that evening, I was beside myself. Already worried about Adeline in the hospital, I somewhat irrationally fantasized all the bad things which could have happened to the children and our friends. I knew I couldn't sleep, so in the blackness of the African night, I drove our rental car nearly a hundred miles to the park entrance. The gate was closed and the registry didn't indicate that our party had left the reserve. After waiting at the exit until nearly daybreak, I drove back to Makumira and found that everybody was back safe and sound. By that time our friends were worrying about my disappearance. They had experienced car trouble and were riding in another vehicle which I did not recognize.

The children excitedly related the details of their scary encounter with an elephant at Amboseli. The van in which the entire group was riding was parked at the foot of a small observation hill in the park. All nine children climbed to the top of the knoll where they enjoyed a vista which included many animals. As they were noisily walking back down, a one-tusked, bull elephant feeding nearby became excited. He charged directly at the children. Some of them ran back up the hill and the others rushed screaming down to the safety of the van. The driver stepped on the starter and raced the engine, diverting the elephant's attention. He broke off his charge a few feet away from the children and backed away. Somebody commented that several guardian angels must have been on duty that day.

The following day I was checking out a new camera at Malde's Camera Shop in Arusha. I found myself standing next to a tall exotic young woman garbed in safari clothes. Wow! Where had she come from? She completed her purchase and made her graceful exit with every male eye following her progress. Mr. Malde confided, "That was Elsa Martinelli, John Wayne's costar in the movie Hatari which is being filmed near here." Since returning to America, we have watched that film on several occasions to refresh memories of exciting days in East Africa. We especially liked the sequence of the baby elephants marching through the streets past the Lutheran church and into our favorite Indian grocery store.

After purchasing my new camera, I was anxious to put it to the test. I walked to the open-air market where dozens of Africans displayed their colorful produce on a beautiful sunny morning. I snapped a couple of panorama shots and was immediately surrounded by a crowd of angry merchants. I hadn't asked permission to photograph them and they were all demanding payment. The situation was becoming noisier and more scary for me until a pair of African policemen arrived. They calmed the crowd and rescued me from an unpleasant impasse. And I learned an important lesson: Get permission before you shoot!

Our return to Kiomboi was again delayed because the vehicle repair wasn't completed. Our children were due back in school before we could get them home. We solved the problem by making arrangements for them to ride the bus taking the other MKs (Missionary Kids) from Arusha to Kiomboi. Our three were delighted with that unexpected adventure with their friends.

That weekend we borrowed a car and drove east to two locations at which our family had lived thirty years earlier. We were thrilled by the first unobstructed view of Mt. Kilimanjaro in our three-plus years in Tanganyika. On all of our previous trips, clouds had concealed this highest elevation in Africa. Kibo's 20,000-foot, snow-covered dome glistened in the morning sunshine and Mawenzi's jagged peaks stood sentinel to the east. Veda recounted details of her three-day ordeal of climbing to the top and the excitement of reaching the summit.

Our first destination, the town of Old Moshi, had been constructed by the Germans at the turn of the century and taken over by the British in 1917. I was born in the hospital there, delivered by an English doctor. Mother had shown us pictures of the house in which we lived in 1924 so we had no difficulty in identifying my first Tanganyika home. We found it unoccupied but still in good repair. We didn't have any African guides so had to use our imagination about how our home had appeared years earlier.

On Sunday we attended Swahili services at the large Machame church whose construction my father had supervised nearly forty years earlier. An estimated three thousand neatly and colorfully dressed parishioners filled the sanctuary and made the rafters vibrate with their magnificent singing. The African pastor introduced us at the end of the service as the children of Bwana Hulti. After the service several people came to me indicating that Daddy had baptized them. A pharmacist named Paulo remembered me as a baby and asked about my brother Paul who had been one of his playmates.

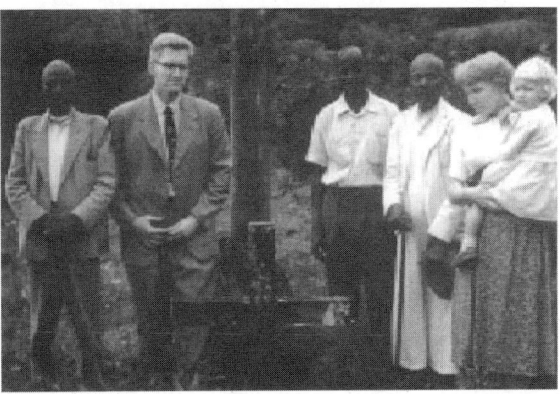

The pastor led us to the nearby cemetery where Veda and I were deeply moved to stand at a burial site marked with a small wooden cross with placard reading, "Ruth Eleanor Hult,1923." Mother had described how this beautiful little sister had died less than twenty-four hours after her birth. Then Mother would declare, "If Ruth had lived we wouldn't have had you, John. Or you would have been a different person than you are."

Years later at Augustana College my brother Paul was excited to meet a woman exchange student from Machame who had walked by this cemetery every day on her way to primary school. She had felt so sorry for this little Ruth lying there all alone that she often brought flowers to place on the grave.

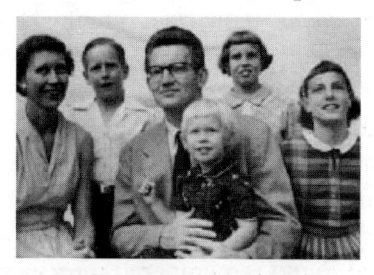

Family photo, 1960

On the following morning, our vehicle was repaired and we were able to return to Kiomboi. Our safari went smoothly, thus ending our final vacation in Tanganyika with many cherished memories of a special segment of our lives.

35. SUNDAY MORNING MEMORIES

Many of my special memories of our days in Tanganyika originated on Sunday mornings. The worship services and other activities associated with that day represented the high point of the week for the Africans and missionaries alike. Over the years our family worshipped in a wide variety of settings ranging from tiny primitive mud hut chapels to attractive brick structures large enough to accommodate over a thousand people. Some of the most meaningful services were conducted out-of-doors. On several occasions we worshipped with congregations of more than five hundred gathered in the shade of a majestic wild fig tree. Other poignant recollections come from Sunday evening services in English celebrated with our mission family and the children at Kiomboi School.

Music was very much a part of African worship and began long before the formal services. The parishioners often had to walk many miles to get to church. If a number of people were moving along together, one leader would chant a theme which would then be echoed in harmony by all the rest. Often these spontaneous hymns would be totally original, with the leader making a statement or exclamation of praise which would then be confirmed and proclaimed musically by his or her companions. At other times they would sing songs with which we were familiar. The beauty and richness of their singing reverberated across the countryside for great distances. This same format was an integral part of their daily life. We were frequently delighted to hear Iramba men, women, and children sing as they cultivated their crops, built their roads, washed their clothes, or pounded their grain. Each of life's activities had its own special rhythm and melody.

When the first German Missionaries came to the Iramba Plateau about a century ago, they brought their hymns and translated them into Swahili and Kiniramba. The Africans learned to sing them and became fond of those which had snappy rhythms and colorful tunes. On the other hand, they distinctly preferred their own indigenous antiphonal music. Asking the Africans to adopt the staid European hymns was akin to requesting a jazz or blues musician to play only classical music. They could do it very well but it wasn't their first love. By the time we got to Tanganyika, the Africans were being asked to create their own sacred music. We enjoyed hearing choirs perform a mixture of our own classical religious music and their traditional music adapted to spiritual themes. Both types were performed beautifully. The rich heartwarming sounds of that continent's music still ring through my memories.

Rev. Howard Olson spent years compiling and publishing original African songs of praise. Several of these stirring hymns are now included in American worship hymnals so we can sing along with our African brothers and sisters.

The spoken word was important, too. Although the sermons tended to be long, they were never boring even though we couldn't understand all the words. In a society where there was still a high percentage of illiteracy, people seemed to maintain a constant alertness so as not to miss a word. With no written word to fall back on, it was necessary to listen carefully. Having grown up with this oral tradition, the African pastors delivered sermons which were colorfully illustrated and eloquently delivered. The actual biblical stories came out of a culture which was similar to the pastoral society of Irambaland. Parables such as that of the lost sheep were totally relevant to the African who remembered exactly the same experience with his own flock. He, too, had spent anxious hours looking for lost sheep, goats, or cattle.

As I sat in church, I was so intrigued in watching those around me that my attention was often diverted from the message. This was not true of the Africans. They hung onto every word and could tell you at the end of the sermon just what the pastor had said.

The congregational seating arrangement found all the men on the right and the women with children on the left. The pews usually consisted of narrow backless benches. As a concession to the missionaries, chairs were often placed in front. We tried to indicate that we didn't want such special treatment but we did prefer to sit together as a family.

The Sunday morning offering format was quite different from what we had experienced in America. In a culture which functioned largely on a barter economy, most people had little or no cash. Worshippers placed their offerings in large collection baskets in front of the altar. The most frequent gifts were ears of corn, small bags of millet, handfuls of peanuts, or eggs. Watching the parade of parishioners of all ages march forward to deposit their offerings fascinated our American children. Scattered among the produce in the basket were a few centis, small copper coins with holes in the center so they could be strung like beads.

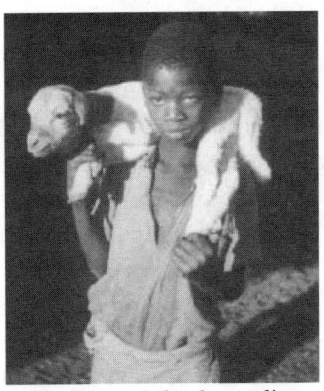

A really special offering might be a live chicken placed in the basket with its feet tied. On one occasion a rooster in the offering basket loosened the knot in a cord around his legs. It flew up into the rafters above the pastor's head. The dedicated clergyman didn't miss a beat as he continued the service. An especially generous gift might be a lamb, a goat, or a calf led or carried into the church and tied to the altar railing. All these offerings were given with total dedication and often real sacrifice. Jesus' parable about the widow's mite certainly applied to all of these humble gifts given by those who had so little.

Other diversions made the African worship services anything but boring. It wasn't unusual for a dog to wander into the open door of a church during a service. The innocent canines were usually evicted by the deacons in short order. At one service I looked up and watched in horror as a big black snake moved from one rafter to another in the direction of a swallow's nest in the highest corner of the church. Apparently everybody else was listening to the sermon for I seemed to be the only person to spot this creature. I was immensely relieved when the serpent became alarmed and disappeared.

Perhaps the most humorous Sunday morning diversion occurred during a baptismal service at Iambi. About a dozen Iramba couples gathered around the altar in front of the church with their babies who were to be baptized. The quiet dignity of the service was rudely interrupted by the hunger cry of one of the infants about four months of age. The young mother reached for her breast to appease the child, but found herself in a bind. She wore a dress, very likely her wedding gown, with a high neckline and no gaps to accommodate a nursing baby. With a bit of contortion and struggle, she managed to reach in and extract her breast. As she withdrew it from under the tight constriction, she exerted so much pressure that a generous stream of milk arched upwards and outward at least ten feet into the congregation. It headed in the general direction where our children were seated. I can still see Dan holding up his hands to shield himself from this unexpected shower. The crying baby was soon contentedly nursing and the service continued uninterrupted, with full dignity. There wasn't so much as an audible chuckle from the African congregation. I didn't laugh out loud, but for the rest of the service, Adeline said that from time to time my internalized mirth would shake the backless bench on which we were seated.

After the service ended the congregation marched out heartily singing a final hymn. Then another happy ritual began. Everybody sought out family and friends and spent a happy time just visiting and enjoying each other. It reminded me of childhood memories of rural churches in America with everybody visiting outside after the service. Young people used this opportunity to get better acquainted and older worshippers, to get caught up on each other's lives. In a special way, the church was a focal center which helped knit the community together. We Americans felt privileged to be included as a part of this extended family in our home away from home.

36. EPILOGUE

My work as a physician in East Africa terminated abruptly on Nov. 21, 1960. According to my diary, "Just as I was turning over to go to sleep at 10:30, I was hit by a terrible constricting pain in my chest radiating up into the neck." My heart was pounding wildly and I was certain that I was having a heart attack.

Adeline ran to get Dr. Lofstrom whose house was at least a quarter of a mile away. She remembers that she couldn't find a flashlight so she used my little otoscope to illuminate the path so she wouldn't step on a puff adder. Dr. Denny was also concerned that I was having a coronary occlusion. A shot of morphine relieved most of the pain but not the anxiety. I was ordered to stay in bed but, over the next few days, paroxysms of severe pain recurred. Each episode brought real fear that I was living my last moments. A radio message was sent to Dr. Joe Norquist who came over from Iambi. He agreed with Denny that I should be flown to Nairobi for evaluation and treatment.

On Dec. 3rd a Missionary Aviation Fellowship pilot flew me to Nairobi accompanied by Adeline, Martha and Veda. I was still hurting and very depressed. Dr. Winteler, a highly regarded British internist, hospitalized me with orders for bed rest. Over the next two weeks, he conducted an exhaustive work-up which indicated some EKG abnormalities.

Adeline had to return to Irambaland and face the heavy responsibility of packing and winding up all of our affairs. Mother was on hand for her four-month African visit with Veda and our family in East Africa then with Ingrid and family in Cameroon. Her presence was helpful and comforting.

Immobilizing episodes of chest pain continued and brought a sad and demoralizing end to our days in Africa. I had no opportunity to say appropriate farewells to the African friends with whom we had shared our lives at Iambi and Kiomboi.

We flew home the first week of January. I particularly remember an agonizing attack during the hours we waited in the Paris International Airport. During this episode, Lud and Esther Melander each held one of my hands and prayed fervently for my welfare. They were on their first plane trip, flying with us on their homeward journey after forty years in Tanganyika.

When we arrived in Minneapolis we were met by my brother David and sister Mary. They were shocked at how gaunt and emaciated both Adeline and I appeared. I was hospitalized at Bethesda Hospital in St. Paul much of the time over the next four months. I had lost fifty pounds and despaired of ever being able to work again. After a prolonged and painful course of a new experimental chelation therapy, I gradually improved and learned to live with the pain. The mission board doctors indicated that a return to Africa was out of the question. We settled in Aurora, Colorado, and had a full rich life for the next three decades.

Cycles of chest pain continued at unpredictable intervals for seventeen years but didn't keep me from work. On Memorial Day, 1978, I was in such agony that Adeline called an ambulance to take me to the hospital emergency room. There a sharp young doctor labeled me a "mystery patient." He suggested new tests which led to a diagnosis of reflux esophagitis. Medical treatment relieved my symptoms and allayed my anxiety.

Our family circle was completed with Tim's birth in 1962. All of our children attended the public schools in Aurora and then pursued their respective professions. Dan became a respiratory therapist and Tim a computer analyst for a petroleum exploration company. Margaret, Elly, and Martha are registered nurses with university degrees.

During the Colorado years, I worked as a pediatrician in private practice, for the Denver School Health Services, and with the Denver Neighborhood Health Program. The latter service in a low-income Mexican-American community was especially rewarding. For several years we also cared for refugee children from Southeast Asia.

I served on the volunteer faculty at the University of Colorado Health Sciences Center teaching clinical pediatrics. Considerable gratification came with my promotion to Clinical Professor of Pediatrics before retirement.

Adeline and I were actively involved with Amigos de las Americas, a people-to-people public health program. We trained high school and college age volunteers for summer projects in several Latin-American countries. I enjoyed a particularly exciting 1969 immunization project in Honduras which was reminiscent of African experiences.

My service in Africa has added a special dimension to all of my subsequent experiences as a physician. I regret that my service in Tanganyika was so limited but am happy to know that the work goes on through the dedicated service of many African co-workers.